*This book is dedicated to all who
seek adventure by kayak and canoe*

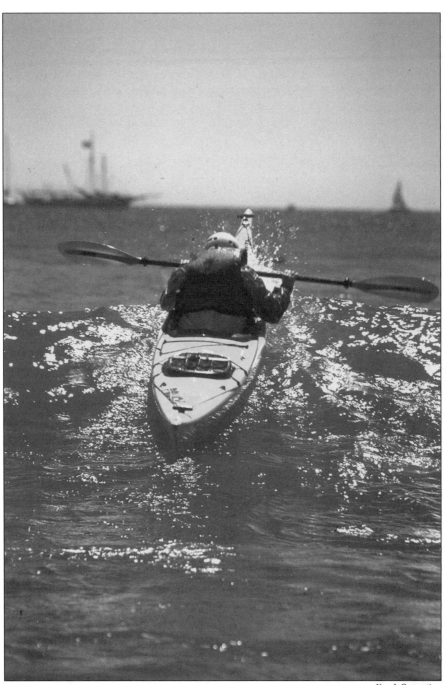

Adventure Kayaking

Trips from the Russian River to Monterey

Includes Lake Tahoe, Mono Lake, and Pyramid Lake

Michael Jeneid

Foreword by Paul McHugh

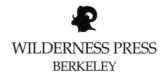

WILDERNESS PRESS
BERKELEY

Copyright © 1998 by Michael Jeneid
Photos by the author except as noted
Maps by the author
Book design by Margaret Copeland—Terragraphics
Front-cover photo: © 1998 by Daphne Hougard
Back-cover photos: © 1998 by Daphne Hougard
Cover design by Larry Van Dyke

Library of Congress Card Number 97-51635
ISBN 0-89997-215-2

Manufactured in the United States of America
Published by: Wilderness Press
    2440 Bancroft Way
    Berkeley, CA 94704
    (800) 443-7227; FAX (510) 548-1355
    wpress@ix.netcom.com

    Contact us for free a catalog
    Visit our web site at www.wildernesspress.com

Front cover: Golden Gate Bridge
Back cover: *top:* Pelicans at Pyramid Lake
     bottom: Osprey on tufa tower, Mono Lake
Frontispiece: Santa Cruz coast (photo courtesy Kayak Connection)

Library of Congress Cataloging-in-Publication Data

Jeneid, Michael.
  Adventure kayaking : trips from the Russian River to Monterey :
 includes Lake Tahoe, Mono Lake, and Pyramid Lake / Michael Jeneid ;
 foreword by Paul McHugh.
    p. cm.
 Includes bibliographical references and index.
 ISBN 0-89997-215-2 (alk. paper)
  1. Kayaking—California, Northern—Guidebooks. 2. California,
 Northern—Guidebbooks. 3. Birds—California, Northern. I. Title.
 GV776.C2J46 1998
 797.1'224'09794—dc21   97-51635
                  CIP

797.1
JEN
1998

Table of Contents

Acknowledgments

I wish to thank my publisher, Caroline Winnett, and editor, Paul Backhurst, for their diligent encouragement and guidance; also Paul McHugh, of the San Francisco Chronicle, for writing the foreword.

Thanks to Carol Jeneid, who steered our Nootka to victory in the Lake Tahoe Outrigger Classic, a 10–mile kayak race, this summer. Her drawing of wildlife at Pyramid Lake enriches this book.

Special thanks to Daphne Hougard, who shares my kayaking adventures. Daphne shot the cover and many other scenes for this book; she has been my coordinator throughout the project, and brought Catherine Sliming, Joanne Coxey and Steve Kasper together to "Shoot the Golden Gate."

My thanks to those of you in the sea kayaking community who have helped me in many ways, especially with your photography. You are all identified with credits for your camera work or in the stories I have told, in which you had your part.

Finally, my thanks to Keith Hansen of Bolinas for contributing his drawing of a spotted owl (Map 5), and to Bill Byrne, way over in Massachusetts, who allowed me to sketch from his humpback whale photograph (Map 15).

Foreword
by Paul McHugh

Kayaking is most essentially a game of balance. Not just in terms of avoiding any tips over into the water—although the majority of kayaks are far more stable than non-paddlers can imagine. The most meaningful balances of the sport are achieved by weighing boldness against caution, by assessing your strengths as modified by your vulnerabilities, and by blending sure knowledge with a willingness to go explore.

In acquiring skill with all these types of balance, a beginning paddler should move warily. Especially, with the last category listed above.

What Huck Finn would have called "book larnin' " is loaded with blind spots. The ideal way to begin in this sport, and to progress in it, is by gaining a bit of basic theory, then some actual experience. Subsequently and sequentially, one should assemble more layers of each. It simply does not do to ignore wisdom of those who have gone before, and just plunge yourself into the wilderness of open water. Nor is it very smart to only take sea kayaking classes and read books, then assume you've got the matter knocked.

That is why this new book from Michael Jeneid is so helpful. Besides tips and lessons, anecdotes and advice, Jeneid presents a full panoply of paddle outings, from outer coastal, to nearshore, to inland sea. The neophyte can pick out mild, sight-seeing tours appropriate for a beginner to do, then read the more dramatic episodes here to glimpse that bourne of adventure which always glitters on the horizon. Even intermediate and expert paddlers can find herein some trip suggestions of which they may be unaware. When was the last time you ran across any explicit directions on how to paddle Pyramid Lake in the Nevada high desert?

Rather than attempt to cover every paddling prospect in the central California environs, Jeneid contents himself with cherry-picking the possibilities. This is not a comprehensive guidebook, but a Whitman's Sampler of outdoor bon-bons. Where the diet starts to grow rich is: first, in the generously detailed directions; second, in Jeneid's artful, hand-drawn maps; third, in the almost offhanded expertise with which he offers wildlife and bird lore for every area; and finally, in the constantly erudite, literate tones in which all of the above is couched.

What I'm attempting to say here is that this book is not just a rather hefty information resource. It's also a pretty darn good read. And a rather unusual one, I might add. Which, in and of itself, is not surprising to me. For as long as I've known him, Michael Jeneid has specialized in the unique.

One of my first memories of him—derived more than a dozen years ago—was acquired at a cross-country ski race at Royal Gorge resort in the Sierra. A crowd of starting skiers vanished across the frozen mere of Van Norden Lake and into the snowclad firs. When they emerged again and drove for the finish line, one person leading the pack was none other than Michael Jeneid. Lean and fit, dressed in a Lycra body suit, he skidded to a stop in a shower of snow crystals, handily taking first place in the Masters division.

Since, one day just previous, I had taken a cross-country ski lesson from him at the Sierra Club's Clair Tappaan Lodge nearby, where he served as chief instructor, I was mightily impressed. Here was somebody who could actually do what he was talking about, and do it rather well.

Years later, as I drove the coast highway past Bolinas Lagoon, I glimpsed a rather trim individual jogging by on the road shoulder. He was lean, muscular, covered in a sheen of sweat. But where he wasn't bald, his hair was greying. "Hmm," I thought. "Seems kinda fit for an older guy. Must work at it." Then my car drew abreast, and I saw clearly who this inspirational individual was: Michael Jeneid.

Many times since, our paths have crossed, and sometimes, our swords. Michael has a strong mind, wide-ranging experience, and firm opinions on most topics—which this former Royal Marine commando is not shy about expressing or defending. Yet, as long as you can defend your own point-of-view against his onslaught in any debate, you will find him a fair and generous antagonist.

The reason why I bring any of this up is simply because, in this book, you will find revealed not only fruits of the labors of one who insists on performing hands-on research, but also a glimpse of the spirit of a man who has pretty much always lived life on his own terms. And I believe that this quality shines through the text. When, I ask you rhetorically, was the last time you ran into someone who can not only provide the natural history of a bird winging or singing overhead, and also, in the same breath, tell you what Chaucer and Shakespeare had to say about it?

In his person and personality—as well as this writing—Jeneid champions the art of honing your body and mind as instruments for being-in-the-world. As a bonus, he thoroughly demonstrates as well that particularly British facility for brandishing eccentricity with panache. Ladies and gentlemen, can you imagine someone paddling across the English Channel whose sole companion on this adventure is a golden hamster residing in a biscuit tin? I rest my case.

So, crack these covers and enjoy yourself! Better still, acquire a kayak and some skills, and launch yourself off in Michael Jeneid's wake, on some of these excellent voyages. You won't be sorry you did.

Introduction

Shooting the Golden Gate

When I told a friend the title of my book is *Adventure Kayaking: Trips from the Russian River to Monterey*, he said: "You're on target! What you need now is a good cover shot." That got me thinking about an image that would link the elemental adventure of kayaking with the advantages of civilization—a hook to persuade people to pick up the book. This is how "Shooting the Golden Gate" became both the cover and the introduction to *Adventure Kayaking*.

For many of us who kayak in Northern California, the most symbolic link between the sea wilderness and civilization has to be the Golden Gate Bridge. There it is, suspended high above the ocean, from two towers—twin pillars of enterprise—defining the entrance to San Francisco Bay. And what are photographs of kayakers framed by bridges for, if not to define our connection with civilization? For me and my friends, how we spend our recreational time defines the quality of our lives. We can go over the bridge to work, and under it for fun.

It's February 23, and four of us in three kayaks are getting ready for a photo shoot with Daphne Hougard, our photographer. The day is brilliantly clear and cold, with strong winds that we hope will fade by the time we meet at Horseshoe Cove—on the southeast side of the Marin peninsula. We'll be using the last hour before sunset to get the best lighting; so, by the time we're in our kayaks, it's 4 P.M. The light is great, but the wind is even stronger than before. It is positively howling.

Daphne has to follow us out under the bridge in a tugboat, using it as a platform for her work. We could have postponed the shoot, but it wasn't easy to get the boat at all, and she'd managed a special rate for the two-hour Sunday shoot.

We hated to give that up. So, when most people are heading home from their weekend fun, we're "outward bound" into the Pacific Ocean on an ebbing tide, buffeted by a wind that will rattle Force 6 on the Beaufort Scale before we're through. The Coast Guard might advise us to go home if they knew which way we are heading. They keep two rescue boats in Horseshoe Cove, and have rescued a few kayakers in the past. We'd like to use their restrooms before we set out, but that's not allowed, and there are no public ones available.

Without our good, oceangoing craft and strong paddlers, this evening's adventure could come apart. As it is, we'll be stretched nearly to the limits of our kayaking skill and stamina, all in the space of two hours. Catherine Sliming is paddling a Sea Cobra, and seaworthy it had better be. As for Catherine, she's been a member of the Canadian National Kayaking Team, both as a flatwater racer and as part of their Dragon boat crew. She's also an R.N. and a pocket dynamo who loves a little offshore action.

Our parent boat is a two-seat, 22-foot uluxtux originally designed for hunting. *Uluxtux* is the Aleut word for the kayak known also by its Russian name, *baidarka*. Steve Kaspar handcrafted it; a blacksmith, he is as strong as two horses and a great offshore paddler with many nautical miles under his stern. With his partner, Joanne, paddling from the bow, they are at home in a rough chop. Their kayak can be driven a long way at five to six knots with this crew. It is the most elegant kayak in use in the Bay Area, and, like the great bridge that will soon be towering over us, it is supremely functional.

Our coordinator and photographer, Daphne Hougard, is a fine kayaker, too. She is the only woman, paddling a single-seat kayak, to have completed the original rough-water ocean race from Fort Cronkite to the Golden Gate, and back, put on by the intrepid Tsunami Rangers. She raced that epic event in heavy seas, using the same boat that I'm paddling this evening. I am the fourth person in this team, paddling an Arluk IV; I should be able to stay upright in this wicked wind. There is no more stable kayak for today's conditions than a "Necky" (the trade name for kayaks designed by Mike Nekker in British Columbia) Arluk IV; its performance pretty well matches that of the other Canadian boat, Catherine's Sea Cobra.

The sky is California blue without a blemish; the sun is in the right place for Daphne's camera; the wind is powerful enough to flatten the water, and erratic enough to hit us from any direction as it comes spoiling along the cliffs and under the bridge. It's the only thing that can cross the path of the sun without casting a shadow. And it can ambush you. (Mark Twain said you should leave the weather out of it because it spoils a good story, but he wasn't a kayaker. For kayakers, weather is usually a large part of the story.)

Daphne's tugboat stands off the boat ramp in Horseshoe Cove as we lever ourselves into our kayaks and quickly raft up. She gets a shot of the three boats locked and sailing like a kayak galleon out of the cove before we break off to head for the bridge. Within minutes, both Catherine and I know we're not tight enough in our boats for the conditions. Loose legs and a slack body in rough water equate with ski boots too big and bindings too loose on one of Squaw's steep runs. Catherine rafts up with the uluxtux to shorten her stirrups on their adjustable straps, and she soon has them giving her whole body good compression in her boat.

My adjustment is more awkward. I have to slide the stirrup bars off their tracks to move the nuts and bolts on them. The water's too rough for me to manage this, but I think rafting up again is too complicated because by now our kayaks are far apart. So I head into the north shore and seek shelter behind a huge rock outcrop, where I find low ledges covered with seaweed. Raising my rudder first, I make a neat seal landing and pull myself well onto a ledge. So far, so good. Off with my spray skirt, left stirrup bar in hand, fingers twiddling the nut, when along comes a sneaky, swelling wave around the back of my rock shelter. It sweeps me off my ledge. A few quick moves, a little luck between the jagged rocks, and I'm back in open water—with no control of my rudder. But Steve and Joanne quickly paddle their stable craft over to me. We make a tight raft and I organize the compression needed to handle the rest of the trip.

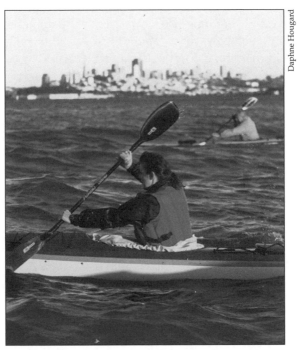

Catherine Sliming and the author beating their way into
San Francisco Bay

The sea pours out of San Francisco Bay as inexorably as sand pours from the top chamber of an hourglass (only this hourglass needs six hours to run out). First it trickles, then it pours unabated until it's done. (Six hours later, on the flood tide, the Pacific Ocean gains ascendance, and back it flows.) We're on our way, and already three solid knots of the ebbing tide are sucking us out to sea. Too soon—before we're ready for it—the bridge is over our heads; high above us we hear the roar of traffic that we can't see, and then we're beyond the bridge and into the open ocean, with a marauding wind for company. The sea here is becoming uncannily agitated yet waveless. One kayak's bow wallows in a trough that gave no sign of its development, while another points its bow up in the air, leaving its stern in the trough. The third kayak misses the hole in the water and surges forward. We have difficulty staying together, partly because the uluxtux is much swifter through the water than the single kayaks, and partly because we are unaccustomed to paddling so close to each other. We've never paddled as a team before.

Daphne takes the tug well ahead of us, goes about and shoots as we get close to her. Closing in on her and staying tightly together isn't easy. With the water moving us around, we collide and clash. We break free, trying to stay close and, at the same time, trying not to run over each other as we set up for each shot. And while we concentrate on getting it right, the tide is sweeping us out to sea.

"Cormorant devouring time" flies by. Already the optimum light is gone and we are a full mile up the coast. We must turn around and get back before dark. Easier said than done! The tug's skipper, Steve Vivello, tells Daphne, "The wind's up to 35 miles per hour; the tide's running full bore at four knots." Daphne's two hours on the tug are going fast.

Going about in the kayaks is difficult, almost unmanageable, with the ebb meeting the wind and the wind just waiting for us to get broadside to it. We are immediately scattered as each one of us tackles the challenge of going about without capsizing in what has become a rambunctious sea. I use several quick, powerful cross-draw strokes, right up at the bow. These strokes are far more effective than sweeping and ruddering, though more risky in rough water than the conventional methods. Now the challenge of getting back— under the bridge and into the Bay—is real. I don't see it as dangerous, yet. And that's good because I didn't come out here for a scare, I just wanted Daphne to get a few, good camera shots. But I'd ask myself, "If I am sitting in the eye of my kayak, sharp as a needle, how many stitches will it take me to sew my way back to Horseshoe Cove?"

The wind is all over the place, blasting hard and then pausing momentarily. But these are false lulls before more violent gusts come from another direction. The near-knockout blows come offshore from the cliffs and hills, generated by the land's shape, causing wind tunnels that concentrate the energy down to the sea's surface. This is how the turbulent areas offshore, known as potato patches, are created. Right now, our three kayaks are in a huge potato field; there's no way we can keep together or help each other.

Steve and Joanne are cutting across the waves ahead of me, while Catherine and I have to butt through them in our shorter kayaks. Their ulux-tux looks superb in the water, with four blades (they are using racing wings rather than conventional paddles) driving their long, sleek hull like a sea lion chasing fish. Catherine is somewhere behind me, and there's no way I can even keep sight of her in this sea if I'm to stay upright. *Sauve qui peut* (save yourself) is the order of the hour. At some point the tug is close enough for me to yell to Daphne, "Stay with Catherine." Dropping back to do this, she gets some great shots as the Canadian drives her Sea Cobra home, under the cliffs against the racing tide. My favorite shot from this trip is of Catherine close to the cliff, ripping into the four-knot peak of the outpouring tide (that's 4.6 mph against her) with a western gull, tucked safely out of the wind, watching her go by. Daphne got me, too, putting in a low brace to survive one of the offshore blasts of wind.

It's a deep dig for all of us, though Joanne and Steve have it made in his incredibly seaworthy craft. They get back under the Golden Gate and turn the corner for Horseshoe Cove well ahead of Catherine and me. We are fighting our way up to the bridge—she can see me, though I can't see Catherine at this point—and we are stuck. Exerting every ounce of strength and skill we have, we try to break out of the jet stream of tide that refuses to let us into the bay. I'm opposite a big rock and mark my progress by it, applying every fiber of muscle in me, while trying to finesse my strokes. What seems like ten minutes goes by before I treat myself to another look. There is no treat. The rock is exactly where it was when I first checked my position against it. The first flicker of failure penetrates my mind, and I know that I can't keep this up much longer. How's Catherine doing? I trust her, but I'm frightened for her. If I'm running out of strength, what's happening to her? The tugboat can pick her up.

"Fear is like fire; it can burn your house down, or you can cook with it!" (Gus Damato said that to one of his fighters.) I'm hungry to get to a safe place, so I cook with it. I'm rewarded almost immediately as the tug chugs past me and Daphne shouts, "You're doing great! Catherine's fine, she's not far behind you." Daphne becomes our coach as we slog it out, gaining water yard by yard. The wind is still pushing Force 6, when a series of running waves that don't break (they just keep rolling along) give us an opportunity. Catherine and I both change our heading to get the best out of the waves, and finally I see her as we surf them right into the Bay. We've done this before, right here.

Only last fall, Catherine in the Arluk IV, Daphne on a Futura surf ski, and I in the Arluk II paddled down from Duxbury Reef out of Bolinas Lagoon to

Horseshoe Cove. In a sea that was very rough—especially right under the bridge—we surfed home past one of the Coast Guard cutters, which was rescuing a capsized catamaran. When we beached in the cove that day, I helped a fisherman get his unruly boat up to the boat ramp. He asked, "Didn't I see you off Muir Beach?" I told him he was right, and he added, "That's some haul in this sea." So I told him that was only half our route, that we'd come 14 miles down from Duxbury in it, and he just shook his head.

It's amazing how much past experience you call on and how much new experience you acquire when you challenge yourself by taking on something difficult. I could have postponed shooting the Golden Gate because of the wind. It was perhaps the sensible thing to do. But, as a famous mountaineer once said, "If you want to climb something worthwhile, at least start." I have some great photos to remind me of that day while I write the less-athletic chapters of *Adventure Kayaking*.

Chapter 1

The Kayak

"Kayak" is the Inuit word for "the man's boat, the small boat, the hunting boat," and "umiak" means "the women's boat, the large boat, the support boat," the boat used to follow the hunters in their kayaks. And so we have identities traditionally attributed to these two unique craft. They were designed and built from the materials available in the Arctic waters where they would be used by the Inuit, "The People."

The raw materials for kayak frame construction were bones of whales, ribs of walruses and narwhals, and driftwood from shipwrecks. Over these strong, flexible frames, sealskins were stretched and sewn together with gut from the same animals whose bones furnished the frames and skins. Paddles were carved from major bones, or from driftwood planks and oars, which helps explain why the surface area of the paddle blades was neither large nor offset, as it can be today. The Inuit hunter was in no hurry: stealth was the key to hunting, not speed. The small boat was built to fit the man who was going to use it, and in some regions, Greenland in particular, it was double-ended so that both the word "kayak" and the look of the craft formed palindromes. Kayaks were always long and lean for easy momentum and quiet glide, but not all the designs were entirely symmetrical and referred to as double-ended; the uluxtux on the cover of this book is a fine example of a design that isn't.

The larger boats followed the hunt, bringing up victuals, replacement hunting gear, dry gear, and morale—anything needed to keep things going at sea as long as the hunt was worthwhile. They carried as much meat from the kill as they could ferry back to their camp while the hunt proceeded, and the rest when it was over. The important thing to understand was the high level of synergy needed for "The People's" survival. And teamwork is still important today.

All the boats called kayaks have this in common: a two-bladed paddle is in the user's hands, to power the craft through the water with alternate strokes on either side of the kayak. (An exception is the King Island Inuit; they paddle with a single blade.) What matters is this: kayaking offers adventure at every level of participation primarily because you have this feeling of independence and control. Being on the water, doing it yourself, you and your boat become a unit. You are the human component in control of a kayak, with your paddle in hand.

Modern Kayak Designs

The sport of kayaking has caught on in a very big way in the past five years, and there are many designs of kayak being used that are quite safe even when paddled by an absolute beginner. These "cockleshell" kayaks are safe for playing close offshore, so long as you wear a life jacket. These kayaks are molded out of plastic materials; almost all are indestructible yet lightweight. They won't sink or even swamp because they are their own self-bailing flotation devices; you sit *on* them, not *in* them. If you are washed overboard you can climb right back on again, so they are a lot of fun for children and inexperienced adults. The best known and widest range of these craft is marketed all over the world under the commercial title, Ocean Kayaks.

Another style of kayak, closer to the real thing because you sit in it and wear a spray skirt to keep the paddle drippings out of your cockpit, is the very small and maneuverable Kiwi Kayak. This craft and its companion two-seater, the Mark Twain, are so stable that it's almost impossible to capsize one; but if you do, it can be brought up with an Eskimo roll. I taught a rolling clinic for Anne Dwyer, the designer (and dean) of these kayaks; it was extremely difficult to turn her Kiwis over in order to demonstrate the roll. Anne's small double kayak, the Mark Twain, is an excellent birdwatching boat; it is small enough for older people to unload from the car and put in the water. It is comfortable, too, with plenty of room for stowing a day pack. With proper care, it is extremely durable.

There is an ever-increasing demand for long, fairly narrow, elegant kayaks that replicate some of the most beautiful craft originally designed by the Inuit. These are marketed by numerous companies as traditional sea kayaks, or touring kayaks. They are beautiful, sleek boats made for a wide range of uses, including camping trips and touring in open water areas, such as the Inside Passage in Alaska, or the San Francisco Bay. The best of them are paddled by elite kayakers in long-distance ocean events. A stable, single-seat, 15-footer, made from plastics, costs about $800. Kayaks built with fiberglass or kevlar are likely to be longer and narrower, and therefore less stable; these will be much faster boats in the right hands (for whom momentum is stability), and cost up to $2,600. Each year in October, most rental programs sell off the kayaks they intend to replace for the next summer. This is your opportunity to pick up a good buy, a forerunner of your "dream boat." The fastest kayaks of the traditional ocean class will be as much as 20 feet long with a 20-inch beam, such as a Necky Luksha II. Paddling this Luksha in the open sea is for a skilled kayaker what a skilled driver must feel when taking a Lamborghini out on the autobahn—the difference being there is no one to crash into and one can roll without getting hurt.

Getting Started

How do you go about becoming a real kayaker, paddling a traditional sea kayak? You sit in—not on—one of these kayaks; though the long surf ski that you sit on is an exception worthy of classic kayak status because of what you can do with it. Given that we're now considering a narrow boat with an enclosed cockpit in which you sit, with a close-fitting spray skirt to keep the water out, there is need for some skill development, including learning emergency drills. You don't set off alone in a traditional sea kayak on open water without any previous instruction or reliable companionship. The first time out you should either be with a competent friend, or, if you don't have that sort of support, sign up with one of the good programs available. There are plenty of them operating year round from Tomales Bay to Monterey. (I've listed in Appendix 1 all the programs with which I've had personal contact as an instructor, participant, or observer.)

Most programs feature a wide range of services, starting with "dressing you" for the sport: with a spray skirt (worn like a tutu) that fits over the kayak's cockpit and keeps the spray out of your boat; and a life jacket. Next comes your paddle, chosen to suit your height and arm length. You'll be

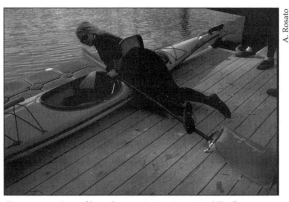

Demonstration of kayak re-entry using a paddle float as an outrigger

shown how to get into your boat, and off you go with your leader for a tour in very safe water. If you want to rent a boat and go alone, program staff will want to know about your competency. Unless they are convinced by your response, you will be encouraged to take a basic class of instruction which will include: paddling technique for forward and reverse movement; turning the kayak with and without use of a rudder; and making a wet exit.

In the primary safety experience, the wet exit, you deliberately fall out of the boat and get back into it by using an inflatable paddle float, then pump the boat dry, and continue paddling. This is one safety class you should take. The second lesson, which is usually the second phase of the same safety class, has you making a wet exit and emptying the boat before reentering it, this time working with a partner whose kayak becomes your support boat. This is the instruction everyone should have taken before setting out on their own

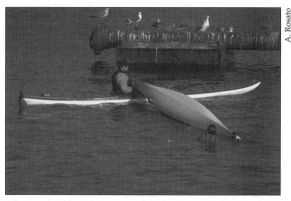

The capsized kayak is emptied by laying it across the deck of your partner's kayak

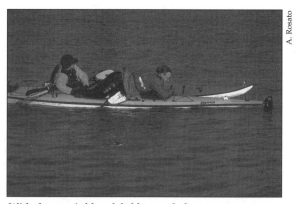

With the emptied kayak held securely by your partner, you can now climb back on board

in a traditional sea kayak. Some people who feel fit and adventurous make the false assumption that kayaking looks easy and so they can't get hurt. Their error is to think they are never going to fall in; when they do it's too late, and they discover they don't have the least idea how to recover.

Trip Preparation

What to Wear: For a day trip you need appropriate hiking clothes for the time of year, and backup clothes and a towel (at least in the car) in case you get wet and cold. In California summer conditions, you must protect yourself from overexposure to the sun. Apart from your face and eyes, which are protected by sunscreen and glasses, it is clothing that serves as the best protection. A long-sleeved shirt or a tank top is good for the upper body, and a cap with a long visor or a wide-brimmed hat is best for the head. Your legs will be under cover while you're paddling, so shorts are okay. Unless you choose to wear neoprene water booties, waterproof sandals, rather than sneakers, are the best footgear. However good the weather, you should always have a wind breaker or warm jersey with you, because water and wind can easily make you cold.

There's a lot of specialized outer clothing you can purchase for kayaking to combat cold, but start with what you probably already own. You might add neoprene gloves to your outfit because, if anything is going to get cold, your hands will. For people with tender skin, kayaking mittens or gloves are useful, year round, to avoid the blisters that easily develop where your paddle shaft fits between forefinger and thumb. If you know you are going to get wet doing safety drills or surfing, you should be wearing either a "Farmer John" (sleeveless wet suit) or a full wet suit at any time of year. Programs that teach wet-exit drills and surfing will either provide a wet suit or ask that you rent one.

Food and Fluids: For a day trip you will need food and fluids; and of these two the fluids are probably more important. Dehydration not only leads to loss of muscle efficiency, but also causes mental depression—not what you want out of kayaking. Drink water regularly throughout the day, and bring a generous supply of it. Natural fruit drinks with their acids and sugar are excellent, and you should often drink whichever you prefer whether you feel thirsty or not. Don't drink alcohol during a paddling trip. Drinking wine or beer with the picnic lunch, unless you've finished paddling, is going to induce fatigue.

Your food choices are unlimited, but a good breakfast is the most important meal for a full day's paddling. A sandwich and fruit for lunch are good, but not too much meat because it's hard to digest while sitting in a kayak. Energy bars are good to eat (you must drink water with these bars for them to be effective) if you are feeling tired on the way home. For longer trips you simply take the same sort of foods you would on a major hike, but you carry much more water unless you know you can resupply. And don't forget your fishing license if you want to try fishing for your supper.

Emergency: The things most easily forgotten, or else deliberately ignored, are those that could save you in a real emergency. If something is ignored, the rationale is, "That wouldn't happen to me, therefore I don't need to prepare for it." And the *it* is the unforeseen element concomitant with any challenge; *it* is the thing that can go wrong. When you actually go kayaking, out of sight or sound of those who could help you, you must be prepared. A whistle, an air horn, a flare, a flashlight, a cell phone, a watch, a compass, a paddle float, a pump, a spare paddle and a first-aid kit are some of the things that you should consider taking with you, depending upon where, how far, and with whom you are going.

Some of us who become passionate about kayaking become professionals; we support, equip, teach, and guide those who want to try it. Some of us write a book about it; and I'm basing this one on things I've seen and taken part in while kayaking over the past fifty years. The territorial focus of the book will be on the warm-climate regions I've explored these past fifteen years: from the mouth of the Russian River at Jenner down to Monterey; plus the four lakes in the Sierra where I paddle every year. All the coastal areas that I describe I use year round, while I paddle the mountain and desert lakes only in the warm seasons.

Chapter 2

On Your Own Trip

After taking the wet-exit safety class with one of the professional programs, here is what you need to know and do to enjoy your own trip, alone or with a friend. Going with a friend is definitely advisable at this stage because you can caution and encourage each other. Whatever you face, two are more able to deal with it and ensure each other's safety.

Under good conditions, most of the trips described in this book can be comfortably completed by anyone who has taken my advice so far—obviously you don't head out into the open San Francisco Bay or under the Golden Gate Bridge yet. In adverse weather, all these trips take on quite a different aspect of severity, though some of them can still be done by working carefully with, rather than against, the weather and the tides. Successful kayaking requires understanding and using the forces of the winds and the tides, while coping with the influences of the water, the air temperature, and the sun. Simply paddling the kayak is only a small part of what you need to know. Knowing when, where, and how far you can go is the more significant part.

Working with nature's constant variables, we can't always have ideal conditions at both ends of our day trip for both putting in and coming off the water, but often we can. If we use the tide chart for our chosen location, we get a good start to the day, and often a less tiring finish. The five crucial things to take into account on your trip are: Tide, Tidelog, Wind, Temperatures, and Sun.

The Tide: Be aware of the state and the shifting of the tides in relation to where you are putting in and where you are going. Be aware of the tide's calculated speed in the tide book and what that speed looks like as you watch the water flowing past a bank, a bridge foundation, a moored boat, or a buoy. What does 2 mph or 4 mph look like? (When you walk up the aisle at your own wedding—that's 1 mph. When you take a brisk walk on the road—that's 4 mph.) Do you know if you are capable of paddling against such a flow? You need to know when it's flooding (coming in) and when it's ebbing (going out); and you should know at what time it will be high water, and what time low water. The quality of many routes entirely depends upon which direction you travel and whether you start and finish at the same point. If it's a round-trip (RT) paddle, start out against the stronger element of the day (usually the wind) and let that element bring you back. On a one-way, shuttle trip, choose which end of your route to start from by opting to "go with the flow." But which flow, wind or water? Go with whichever is stronger.

The Tidelog: The Northern California *Tidelog* is sometimes called "the little black book" after its black cover. It is a "must have" for fishermen and boaters of every kind throughout Northern California, published by Pacific Publishers in Bolinas. It describes and illustrates the tides, the currents, the moon (the main determinant of the tides), sunrise, sunset, dawn, and dark. It is a graphic almanac and a work of art, so easy to follow that you need no instruction here on how to use it. It is available at all kayaking stores and many bookshops.

The Wind: Be aware of the wind's direction and force, and I emphasize the word force. Remember that it tends to be absent or mild in the morning and to build up during the day. It can be a terrific help adding to your adventure, or it can quite suddenly become a real danger. Sea kayaks catch a lot of wind and canoes even more; it can be hard work to paddle either craft into the wind over open water, and harder still to paddle across the wind. Paddling across is when you are easily broached, and most likely to capsize. A 15 mph cross- or headwind is about as much as you can face as a beginner, even though the same wind is fine if it's behind you. So the strength and the direction of the wind must always be factors in your decision to go out—or not. There is the internationally used Beaufort Scale of from 1 through 10, for recording the force of the wind (see Appendix 3).

Temperatures: Besides the air temperature of the day, which may be pleasantly warm, the temperature of the water into which you could capsize, or with which at least your hands may be in contact for several hours, is of critical importance. Apart from anything else, it should determine whether to use a wetsuit or a drysuit (one that lets no water make contact with your body), if you are on water from which you cannot immediately make a safe withdrawal to dry land and warmth. The ocean is the most obvious place to be wearing a full wetsuit, or in midsummer a Farmer John; but if there's any risk of total immersion in any cold body of water, wear a full wetsuit. As for the air temperature, the wind is critically important, because of the wind-chill factor. Combine this factor with wetness and you get a double-jeopardy effect.

Wet skin, even in fine conditions, reduces the temperature of what it's covering by an alarming percentage. (This is why driving through deserts in Australia, your drinking water is carried in a big canvas bag outside the truck that has a weave loose enough for its exterior to become saturated. The cooling effect at the bag's wet surface is conducted to the water inside the bag; thus your drinking water is 15 degrees cooler than the air temperature.) Kayakers should be aware that a lovely, sunny day may have a cold wind for company, and anything wet that is exposed to the wind—hands for instance—will soon be chilled.

The Sun: We all want the sun for warmth, for light, for energy, and for all our outdoor activities. For each trip consider where the sun will be in relation to your direction of travel. Decide which direction to travel some routes by putting the sun as near as you can to where you'd most like it to be. It's best to have it over your shoulder for as much of the day as possible; that's a lot easier on the eyes and much better for binocular and camera use. If it's behind you, there's a much better view of everything to be seen, and your face doesn't get cooked by it. Given fair conditions, my direction of travel may be decided by the position of the sun.

Putting in and Hauling out: Having worked out your route for the day, you need a decent spot for getting onto the water as well as for getting off it. This is when you are most likely to damage your kayak, unless you have a soft sand beach at your disposal. Many launching sites have wooden boat docks that are a help, but look out for jagged metal protruding through woodwork and rubbing guards. Nothing worse can tear into your kayak. Concrete slipways are often available, but you must either set up a seaweed slide or place your kayak in the water and enter the cockpit by using your paddle as an outrigger, with one blade braced on the rear deck and the other on the concrete.

Rescues: Self-rescues after capsizing and the Eskimo roll are skills to be learned in a controlled environment. If you are going to become an adventurous, solo kayaker, you'll need to learn rolling techniques in addition to self-rescues. If you are not attempting technically advanced trips, what you learn about rescues in the classes already described will suffice. Rescues in which you do not leave your cockpit after falling are more sophisticated, and would be learned in a more advanced class.

Paddling: Paddling well enough to enjoy yourself without straining muscles is easy as long as you're not going far or not going against the elements. In these cases it doesn't matter whether the two blades of your paddle are offset or in line. In-line paddling will seem less complicated to the beginner; and some programs suggest that their clients start out that way. Yet offset blades allow you a better performance, for at least three reasons. First, the inactive blade cutting through the air offers much less resistance to the wind. Second, subsurface strokes, as used in the Eskimo roll, are blocked by equal and

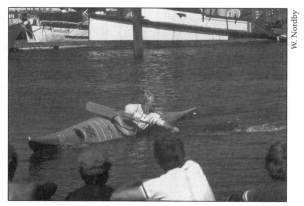

Instructor Derek Hutchinson demonstrates a low-brace turn at Sea Trek

opposite resistance if you don't have an offset, inactive blade. Third, the hand control and the variety of movements involving the shoulders when using an offset blade are in the long run physically more effective.

The spacing between your hands on the paddle is important. If they're too close together, you cannot get any strength into your stroke; if they're too far apart, your stroke becomes clumsy. A good guide is to first hold the paddle horizontal over your head, with your shoulders back and elbows bent. Keeping your hands equidistant from the blades, move them along the shaft until you have a right angle at your elbows. Keep your handholds and bring the paddle down in front of your chest. What you see in front of you is approximately the best position for your hands on the paddle. To make the necessary rotation of the offset blades between strokes, the right hand grips the shaft and causes the rotation. The left hand is allowed to open slightly while the shaft is turning, but it closes on the shaft as you start the stroke on your left side. (This description is for right-handed paddlers; lefties hold firm with their left hand.) The hand that controls the rotating always remains in a closed grip on the paddle.

Good posture in the kayak—without lounging back as if in an armchair— is important. To paddle effectively you must have compression coming from your feet through your braced thighs and your seat that gives your torso a firm base from which to work. Using your shoulders and your back, while slightly rotating from the waist, is part of the technique needed to paddle effectively. Your arms should be braced and only slightly bent, so that they form a triangle with the shaft of your paddle. They should not be going round and round in circles as your legs do when you ride a bicycle. The most effective recreational paddling will be that which takes its basic form from the techniques of the best competition paddlers, like Greg Barton. I'm not suggesting you paddle hard or fast. My technique when bird watching by kayak is the same as when I race. I use the same kayak for both; only my tempo changes as I slow down from 6 to 2 mph.

If you are on a long journey, your decision making about how to deal with the elements remains the same. On each succeeding day, you assess the wind, the tide, the temperatures, and the sun, and you work within these unavoidable variables. They govern your life. Throw in a spell of bad weather as a joker, and you don't have to struggle with that card; take some R & R. Rest up, gain a little strength, explore the beach, or hike inland for a better view of where you're going.

The longest solo journey I ever made took me six weeks; much of it through appalling weather and some of it in horrendous seas that either snuck up on me or found me ambitious enough to tackle them. I had a young man's mission: to get from London to Paris to see my girlfriend, on very little money. Without enough funds for trains, ferrys, hotels and restaurants, I did acquire a canvas kayak built by Mr. Herschfelt of Twickenham, 20 miles above Westminster on the River Thames. My down payment of five pounds (worth $20 then) left me just enough cash to buy tea, rice, powdered soups, and hardtack.

That was in 1957. I had fifteen pounds to live on and reach my destination in six weeks. I neither knew how long it would take me to get from one place to the next, nor where the next place would be because I'd never done this before, and was learning how to do it as I went. I did not know about offsetting my paddle blades, but I could follow a compass. Success each day depended on the tides, the wind, and the weather (there was a lot of rain). I tried to gauge these elements each day at dawn, and except when the weather stopped me cold, or a squall at sea washed me ashore, I combined tuition with intuition until I got there.

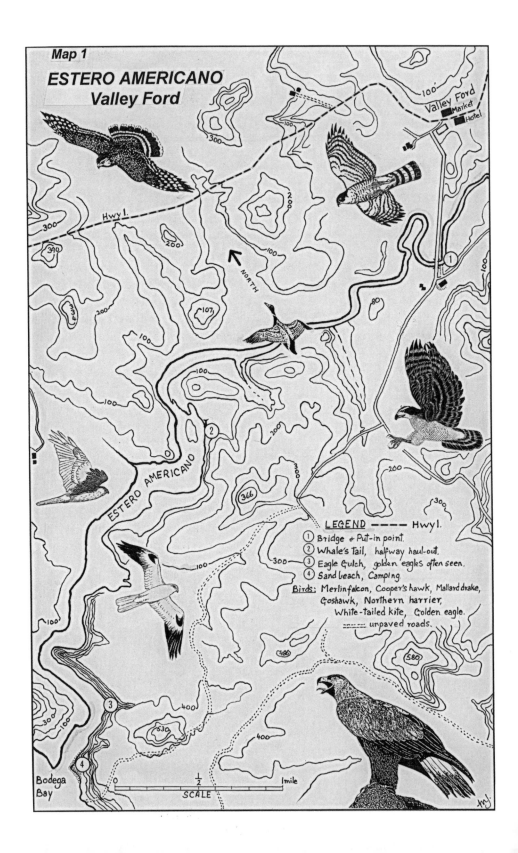

Map 1

ESTERO AMERICANO
Valley Ford

Valley Ford
Market
Hotel

Hwy 1.

NORTH

ESTERO AMERICANO

LEGEND ———— Hwy 1.
① Bridge & Put-in point.
② Whale's Tail, halfway haul-out.
③ Eagle Gulch, golden eagles often seen.
④ Sand beach, Camping.
Birds: Merlin falcon, Cooper's hawk, Mallard drake,
Goshawk, Northern harrier,
White-tailed kite, Golden eagle.
------- unpaved roads.

Bodega
Bay

0   ½   1 mile
SCALE

Chapter 3

North of Tomales Bay

TRIP 1 ESTERO AMERICANO:
Valley Ford to Bodega Bay

Type	Length	Map
Moderate day	12 miles RT to Bodega Bay	1
Easy overnight	12 miles RT to Bodega Bay	1
Easy day	6 miles RT to Whale's Tail	1

Summary and Highlights

The trip is 6 miles (one way) from the put-in point at the bridge 1 mile south of Valley Ford, down to the ocean in Bodega Bay. It is a shallow-water route of outstanding pastoral beauty. Sand dunes inside the ocean beach destination offer wind protection for camping out. It is an easy trip, as long as you work with wind and tides. There is a good, halfway haul-out point at the Whale's Tail for those who want a shorter, relaxing trip. The estero is a riparian corridor in which many species of raptors hunt on their migration and others breed; it is also frequently visited by white pelicans. The Point Reyes Tule elk herd roams over the high ground where the estero approaches the sea, and white-tailed deer often browse close to the water.

Special Advice

Do not go to this estero without checking your tide book. The first 3 miles are always navigable, but at low, low tides there is not enough water to get you much farther. When winter storms seal the mouth of the estero, it fills up with enough drainage water to be navigable all the way to the sea. Since there is no tidal ebb or flow then, you can paddle down and back at any time of day. In late March or early April when the estuary opens up, the sea bass can get in and out again, and you must become tide conscious again.

Unless you are a very competent ocean paddler you should not commit yourself to navigating the fast outflow of water from the estero into Bodega Bay. When you reach the last lagoon, keep to the left and make your landing.

How to Get There

Take Route 101 to Petaluma, 30 miles north of the Golden Gate Bridge. Watch for the E. WASHINGTON ST. CENTRAL PETALUMA sign and 0.75 mile after this sign exit at a smaller sign, BODEGA BAY—BUSINESS DISTRICT. At the light, turn left onto E. Washington. After 1.1 miles, E. Washington becomes Washington, and at 1.7 miles it becomes Bodega Avenue. Stay on this road for 19 miles to Valley Ford. After 17.5 miles, Shoreline Highway (Route 1) joins Bodega Avenue, and the route north, from here on, is called Route 1. Just before taking the uphill, right-hand curve into Valley Ford you'll see a llama farm on your right.

The Valley Ford Market, on your right, is well stocked for putting a lunch together, and there is an outside toilet. (It's the last chance you'll have to use one on this trip.) Across the road from the market is the Valley Ford Hotel (707) 876-3600, an excellent bed and breakfast inn. Next to the market is a small gas station.

The difficult thing now is to find the little lane that leads down to the Estero Americano. From the market, look across Route 1 to your right, where you'll see a restaurant—DINNUCCI'S ITALIAN DINNERS. Drive 100 yards over to it, and you'll see a black-on-yellow road sign directly ahead of you, 15 MPH, with an arrow for a sharp left turn. Forty yards beyond this sign, turn left into the lane, which is unnamed and remains invisible until you turn into it. Go 0.8 mile down this road and cross the bridge over the Estero Americano. As soon as you cross the bridge, turn left onto Marsh Road and immediately left again onto an old road, which takes you down to the water's edge. Park here for the day or overnight, but park considerately to let others to share the limited space. This is your put-in point, right under the bridge, for a few memorable hours in paradise.

Trip Description

The distance from your put-in point down to the ocean is 6 miles; this distance may be enjoyed as a full-day trip there and back, or as an overnight if you sleep down by the ocean and return the next day. There is a third, unhurried, full-day trip for those who want to move slowly to absorb the remark-

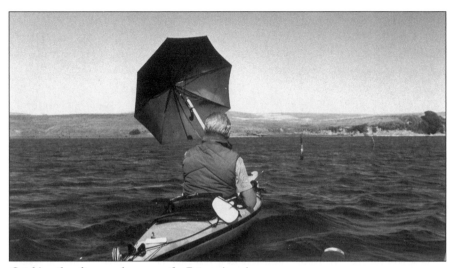

Catching the afternoon breeze on the Estero Americano

able tranquillity of the estero. This trip goes halfway to the ocean, stopping at "the Whale's Tail" (a one-of-a-kind rock whale sculpted by Mother Nature) on the left bank.

The shorter trip is ideal for a family canoe or a kayak trip. Paddle 3 miles in, usually with some wind resistance, and 3 miles out with the strong afternoon wind pushing you home. For the full 6-mile journey, start early and paddle the whole distance to the sea before the wind rises. When you return, the afternoon wind will astonish you with its cooperation, especially if you have a full tide eliminating shallow water drag from your kayak's bottom.

The entire estero is shallow, but it is navigable for the first 3 miles to the Whale's Tail at almost all tides, year round. Where you put in, the estero isn't much more than a wide ditch, and you must head left (west) under the bridge. Look up as you glide beneath this bridge and you'll see that cliff swallows have glued their procreant cradles under its eaves. Meadows on both sides are well above the water level; black-and-white Holsteins and a few horses look down at you from their grazing. As you were putting in, you may have heard the babylike screams of adult red-shouldered hawks that live in the trees around the nearest farm, and you may have seen them; they are resident year-round. Certainly you'll see red-tailed hawks and kestrels throughout the day.

As the estero meanders west it gets wider, and on either bank you are almost bound to see a small, black-and-white flycatcher hawking at insects from old fence posts. This will be a black phoebe or, if it's a bit bigger and brown instead of black and white, it will be a Saye's phoebe. There are many tyrants over insects, swallows as well as flycatchers, hawking over the water.

And there are hunters of fish: kingfishers, occasional ospreys, cormorants, pelicans, and three species of heron. Also, there are hunters of mice, crickets, lizards, and small snakes: the kestrel, the white-tailed kite, and the northern harrier. The list of predators grows even more impressive as you head downstream.

On the left bank, 0.5 mile past the bridge, you'll see a lovely grove of bay trees with masses of white blooms in the early summer, and big green leaves that give excellent cover, year round, to two deadly predators: the Cooper's hawk and the sharp-shinned hawk. These two practice "still hunting" by sitting motionless behind this cover until they see some unwary blackbird, robin, or jay flying across the water. When that happens they rush out and bind to their prey with cruel claws. (Falcons have talons, accipiters have claws.) In the fall, round about early October, there's a good chance you'll see the fiercest hawk of all, a goshawk, come out of these bay trees. It gets its name from being strong enough to kill a wild goose.

You may see all of these things in the first mile, and then as the estero begins to widen and the land opens out, with secondary tree growth on the slopes behind the flats, you are in kite territory. The estero straightens out, widens considerably, and heads due west for the next mile. Now, you'll meet the wind, which hasn't bothered you this far: the later you start out, the stronger the wind. An early start is always a good idea; however, when you return, that same wind is going to be behind you, and on drafty days you can get a wonderful ride back. Egrets (snowy and great), great blue herons, and cormorants frequent this reach; the meadows are now almost at the same level as the water, so that the littoral is a gentle mud slope, and you'll begin to meet shorebirds such as godwits and willets. In winter months, there will always be buffleheads and golden eyes, but these ducks leave in the spring.

After 2.5 miles, the estero takes a left turn, where, on the right bank, you may see a duck blind under a black oak. This could surprise you, but of course the farmers of all this land hunt and fish, and it is certainly their right to do so. In another 0.25 mile you'll have to decide whether to turn left again into what looks like a tributary, or go straight ahead on the main body of water. Take the left turn even though you see water straight ahead, because there is rarely enough water for your passage through this area. Besides, what looks like a tributary is a deeper channel, around a low-lying island of mud and pickleweed, that brings you back to the mainstream.

As you follow this channel, it will curve around to the right, closing on an escarpment on your left, and as you follow this slope you'll see ahead, to your left, a quite remarkable, smooth rock that looks just like a whale's tail tipped up in the air. It's that big. It has a small plateau of grass around it, and it's an ideal spot to take a break, have lunch, or stop. You've come 3 miles so far, and if you want an easy day this may be far enough. You have a lovely, wide expanse of shallow water in front of you where the white pelicans land to fish when they come this way. If they do, you're in luck because they have dropped in for a change of scene from Tomales Bay; they look twice as big as brown pelicans, and are much more sociable birds.

If you decide to paddle on, there's another 3 miles to go before you reach the ocean, and it's certainly worth the effort as long as you're not using the last hours of a falling tide. If you do that, you may get stuck in the mud, particularly in the next quarter mile. Check your tide book! Keep to the left side of the wide section ahead for the next quarter mile and, if the tide is low, follow the line of small branches that are put in by local fishermen to mark the way. If these markers are not visible, stay approximately 75 yards offshore from the left bank. Once you are out of this shallow zone, there's enough water to get you down to the sea, except at a low, low tide.

You are moving now into an area in which surf scoters and scaups are the birds on the water, and in the winter months you are likely to meet that wandering falcon, the peregrine. By now, the country on either side of you is very grand—big, rolling hills, no roads, no telegraph poles in sight, just the occasional farm set well back from the estero, in the hills. But there is the wind again. In the afternoon it's usually strong and right in your face; while it offers some resistance, it doesn't interfere with your heading. Besides, it feels good.

The Whale's Tail is now one mile behind you, and on your left there's a broad bay of shallow water. Don't wander into it unless there's a really high tide, in which case it's worth exploring. It leads you into a creek and fresh meadows, where you may find yellow-breasted meadowlarks, each one singing "with careless happiness, giving its song a try," and shorebirds called greater yellow legs that sound their alarm long before you reach them.

When you are past this bay, the ground on both sides of the estero changes radically; that's part of the beauty of this trip. A steep headland juts out into the water on your left, and you must paddle around it. From here on, the land begins to tower over you with a mountainous effect. Look out for Tule elk on the skyline to your left and keep an eye on the sky itself because this is definitely golden eagle territory. As you follow the water, you enter an L-shaped gorge. It's like navigating in a Norwegian fjord.

It was here that Catherine Hickey, from the Point Reyes Bird Observatory, and I once saw five golden eagles, two adults and three juveniles. The entire family was sky diving around us, using the airstream of a steep gully, at the bottom of which we had hauled out for lunch. We made tea and watched, spellbound for an hour, while these five monarchs entertained us. The foot of this gully is 5.5 miles from your Valley Ford put in, and it's a good haul-out spot if the wind is up, or if you don't have time to get down to the mouth of the estero. I call it Eagle Gulch on the map.

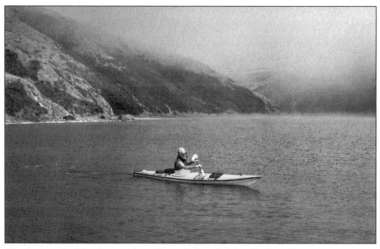

The last pool of the Estero Americano before it joins Bodega Bay

Another half mile to go, and in that half mile you may meet all three species of scoters in the winter months: the black, the white-winged, and the surf scoter. On your left, ahead, there's a wide expanse of sand and dunes beside a final broad pool of water. This pool will either be blocked in by a sand bar from the sea in winter, or will be tidal with a narrow cut through the sand bar, in which case turn left onto the sand flats before you get carried out to sea.

This is a perfect place for camping out of your kayak. You can walk the ocean beach and listen all night to the surf pounding on the shore; the killdeer plovers will echo their name incessantly, "killdee, killdee." And, if you don't see an eagle, you will definitely see and hear that "treble-dated crow" the raven—a bird said by the Greeks to live three times as long as the stag.

The most remarkable thing I've seen on this estero was in midwinter when I was race training on a Futura surf ski, rather than a kayak, and using what's called a "wing" instead of a conventional paddle. Wings are the modern, carbon fiber tool for racing; in the hands of an elite paddler they are considered fractionally better than the best paddles. The idea was to cover the 12 miles, down to the ocean and back, in under two hours. I'd picked a good tide, so that there'd be no drag on the surf ski caused by shallow water, and started early so that the wind wouldn't be a factor. I was zipping along when a bird came out from some old black oaks, ahead of me on the left bank, and started to fly very erratically across the estero.

It was a long way ahead of me and unidentifiable at first. In fact, its identity would not have mattered except that I became aware of a much bigger bird, careering all over the place in the same vicinity, apparently attacking it. Then I realized I was seeing a hawk and its quarry in a frantic tail chase. The hawk was big, and cutting such short, sharp turns in close pursuit of its quarry that I thought it might be a goshawk. But as I closed rapidly, with my own wings flailing the water, I saw that the hawk was so dark that it looked almost black. It was a Peal's peregrine, one of the Pacific coast variety, and I was watching a duel of wits between a wandering falcon and a kingfisher that didn't want to be that pilgrim's dinner.

The two birds, the killer and its quarry, were dodging back and forth low over the water, rather than in a direct line of chase—a race the crafty kingfisher knew it couldn't win. For this reason I was able to close in on the action and stop paddling; and they were oblivious to my presence as I sat there watching. Now, the falcon threw itself high up into the air, rolled over onto its back, like a fighter pilot doing an Immelman turn; then it dropped one long wing so that it pointed down to the water and let its whole body finish the roll and follow that wing. It was such a languid move that the speed of the falcon's flight while performing it was veiled by its elegance. I was witnessing the peregrine's classic "stoop," in delta shape, as it dived at terrifying speed to kill the kingfisher.

Yet, as the falcon's stoop brought it close enough to execute its coup de grace, the kingfisher stopped flying and dived head first into the water, where it stayed long enough to completely confuse the falcon. The peregrine, unable to see what it thought it should have in its grasp, gained height to review the situation, while the kingfisher was winging it back to the bank.

When Pamela Feinsilber, editing a piece called "Elemental Journeys" for San Francisco Focus, *asked me to name the best place for a peaceful paddle out of all the places I go kayaking, I had to say it was the Estero Americano. And when she asked me if there was anywhere out of the ordinary to stay overnight nearby, I had no hesitation in recommending the Valley Ford Hotel (in lieu of the sandbar, where I prefer to sleep down by the ocean). She liked the sound of it so much that she gathered some friends and came to do the trip with me.*

What she might not say is that, not only did we have several close-up views of a green heron on that trip, but the trip leader set fire to his kayak. And so I caution you: if the wind is so strong that you use the cockpit of your kayak to brew up the tea, don't sit down to drink it without turning the stove off!

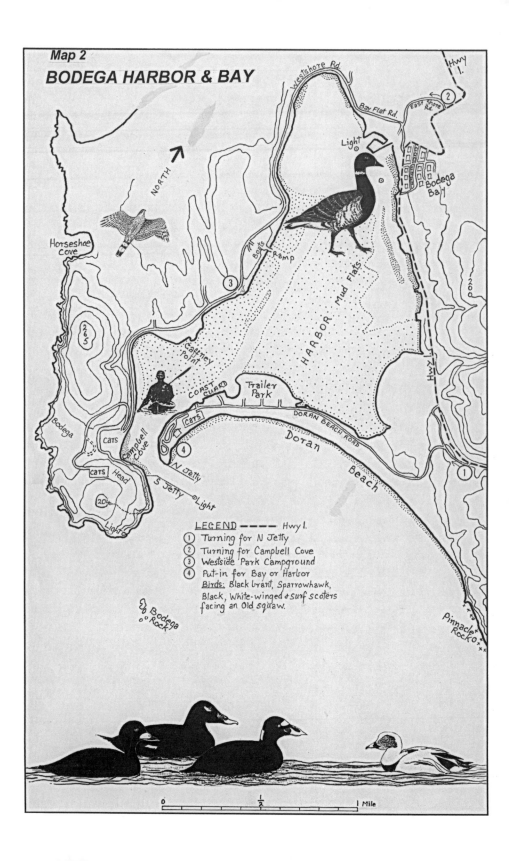

Map 2
BODEGA HARBOR & BAY

Hwy 1.
Westshore Rd.
2
Bay Flat Rd.
East Shore Rd.
Light
Bodega Bay
NORTH
Horseshoe Cove
Boats
Ramp
3
HARBOR Mud Flats
265
200
HWY 1
Cattney Point
COAST GUARD
Trailer Park
DORAN BEACH ROAD
Cars
Doran Beach
Bodega
Cars
1
Campbell Cove
Cars Head
4
N Jetty
S Jetty
Light
204
Light

LEGEND ----- Hwy 1.
① Turning for N Jetty
② Turning for Campbell Cove
③ Westside Park Campground
④ Put-in for Bay or Harbor
Birds: Black brant, Sparrowhawk,
Black, White-winged & surf scoters
facing an Old squaw.

Bodega Rock

Pinnacle Rock

0   ½   1 Mile

TRIP 2   BODEGA HARBOR & BAY

Type	Length	Map
Easy half-to-full-day exploring	2–6 miles	2

Summary and Highlights

This is a harbor exploration trip rather than a journey. Both Bodega Harbor and Bodega Bay, which is the ocean bay off Doran Beach between Bodega Head and Tomales Bluff, are easily accessible from the same two put-in points at the harbor mouth. The put-ins are separated by only 0.2 mile of water, but they are 8 miles apart by road. One is at the North Jetty of the Bodega Harbor mouth, at Doran Park Trailer Park, and the other at Campbell Cove. This cove is just inside the harbor mouth, neatly sheltered behind the inside corner of the South Jetty, and from it you can take an excellent walk up onto Bodega Head. From this vantage the entire harbor to the north, Tomales Bay to the southeast, and the sea-lion colony to the east can be viewed. The entire area is excellent sea-birding territory.

Special Advice

Doran Beach, by the North Jetty, is a good put-in point for day trips, but for an overnight it's well worth driving around to the Westshore campsite close to Campbell Cove. Bodega is the most active professional fishing and recreational boating harbor between San Francisco and Fort Bragg; when in the deep water channel of the harbor, pay attention to all vessels and stay out of their way.

How to Get There

To get to the North Jetty, at Doran Trailer Park, follow directions for Trip 1 to Valley Ford; continue north on Route 1. At 6.7 miles look for S. Harbor Way on your left; it is just before a tight right bend in the road. 50 yards beyond S. Harbor Way, also on the left, is a little road, not named, that winds uphill. It has a hotel sign on it for BODEGA BAY LODGE. Drive up to that sign to put yourself on Doran Park Road. As you draw level with the hotel a small sign confirms that Doran Park is directly ahead. Pay a $3 day fee or a $14 camping fee at the Doran Park ranger hut 0.5 mile ahead. From the hut, drive on Doran Beach Road for 2.5 miles to reach the harbor-mouth parking lot and beachhead, facing southeast to Tomales Bay. You can see all the way down to Hog Island in Tomales Bay, 12 miles southeast of the Bodega Harbor mouth.

At the North Jetty, Doran Park Trailer Park offers 128 trailer sites and 10 tent sites. For tents, this is a very windy area that I do not recommend; you will do much better to camp on the Campbell Cove side of the harbor, at Westside Park Campground.

To get to Campbell Cove and Westside Park Campground drive north on Route 1 from the junction with Doran Park Road, through the town of Bodega Bay. It will help to set your odometer at zero as you pass the Route 1 junction with Doran Park Road. At 1.2 miles a 76 gas station is on your right. As you leave the town, at 2.15 miles, follow the sign for BODEGA HEAD—WESTSIDE PARK MARINAS. Turn left onto East Shore Rd. Drive downhill 0.3 mile and turn right onto Bay Flat Rd. At 2.8 miles Bay Flat Rd. turns right, but you follow the bay shoreline on what is now Westshore Rd. A large parking area on waste land is on your right at this junction. You can put in for a day trip from this lot, but it's well worth continuing to Campbell Cove. Continue on Westshore Rd. past Spud Point Marina at 3.65 miles. Go past Westside Park Boat Launching Facility at 4 miles and, immediately after it, turn into Westside Park Campground if you want to camp. If not, keep going. At 5.4 miles you reach Campbell Cove, where there is free day parking and a good put in from the sandy cove just below the parking lot.

Trip Description

Bodega Harbor is a lagoon waiting to be explored; it's 2 miles long, north to south, and almost 2 miles wide at its broadest. It is protected from the open sea of Bodega Bay at its southern end by the slender arm of a mile-long sand spit, the seaward side of which is Doran Beach. To the west it is protected by high ground, over 200 feet in elevation, forming Bodega Head; and where the sand spit and the headland nearly meet are two riprap jetties. These are North and South Jetty, guarding the entrance to the harbor's sanctuary. The harbor has a 2-mile, deep-water channel, running north to south, and more deep water throughout the northerly 0.5 square mile. The remaining 1.5 square miles of the area is very shallow; it becomes an extensive area of sand and mud flats at low tide.

The harbor is the most active boating area between San Francisco and Fort Bragg, and it has a large professional fishing fleet as well as a Coast Guard station. We kayakers need to be aware of our nuisance potential to boat skippers, who have limited water in which to navigate without error. They have to stick to the deep channel, which gets them from the harbor mouth up to the town of Bodega Bay and the Westside Boat Ramp. In our kayaks we are very small, and though we have plenty of room to move around, we are often slow in doing so. Pay attention to the movement of bigger craft, especially fishing boats, whose skippers exercise a strong imperative in matters of right of way.

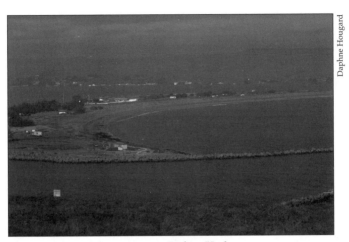

Doran Beach and the entrance to Bodega Harbor

The real Bodega Bay is part of the ocean, a 6-mile coastal indentation from Bodega Head down to Tomales Bluff, at the entrance to Tomales Bay. The northwest end of this bay is well sheltered in the crook of the Doran Beach sandspit down to Pinnacle Rock, 2 miles east of the North Jetty. This 2-mile stretch of the coast is a perfect place for an entry-level, ocean kayaking experience, provided you stay inside the natural boundary circumscribed by a line drawn from Bodega Head through Bodega Rock (a half mile east of the headland) to Pinnacle Rock. Pinnacle Rock stands out like a tufa tower, close to shore off the east end of Doran Beach.

This 2-mile zone of calm water has one possible drawback: sharks. Great white sharks are a factor to consider when offshore kayaking down this entire coastline. However, I spend a lot of time making offshore journeys and accept the danger as somewhat less than that of driving on any street in any city. There are more deadly drivers clinging to their car phones behind the wheel in the Bay Area than there are deadly sharks wheeling around in Bodega Bay. There are two primitive ways of dealing with one's fear of sharks when traveling offshore: keep moving quite fast because they prefer a stationary target; once in a while smack the water very hard with the flat blade of your paddle. This makes a sharp, offensive noise that may deter sharks from investigating you.

The two put-in points for starting your offshore adventure at Bodega are the same two you use for exploring the harbor: Doran Beach and Campbell Cove. Campbell Cove is a delightfully sheltered little cove, from which you can put in from a firm sand base at low tides; it has a free, day-use-only, parking lot right behind it. From here you can look straight out between the two harbor-mouth jetties down to Pinnacle Rock, or survey most of the harbor to your left. If you want to go out into the bay, it's a 0.25 mile paddle to clear the

North and South jetties. A left turn will put you into Bodega Bay alongside Doran Beach.

A road runs from the cove uphill onto Bodega Head. If you walk this road, going left where it forks, you'll come to a parking lot. From this lot several trails lead you toward the ocean. The views are outstanding, especially south, to the sea-lion colony on a harsh island of rocks; and the whole headland is occupied by that little gem, the American goldfinch. At low tide you can follow a path down to the South Jetty to make your way back to Campbell Cove along the shoreline. Do not go out onto the jetty: there is a sign forbidding access.

If you want to explore the harbor, at low tides you paddle a half mile northeast across the harbor to the Coast Guard Station and turn north from there. You'll be in the deep channel that takes you the 2 miles up to the harbor, and you'll find plenty of deep water in all directions there. At high tide, you can paddle almost anywhere you please, all over the harbor. And there is much to see.

Other Options

Leaving from Campbell Cove or Doran Beach, as already stated, looking southeast you can see all the way down to Hog Island. It's 12 miles away, and it makes a great offshore trip if you're a hard-core ocean kayaker. You must realize, if you go any distance at sea beyond Pinnacle Rock toward Tomales Bay, you are "out of bounds" unless you are an expert sea kayaker. You will no longer have a soft-sand lee shore on which to rest if you get tired. You will no longer be in sight or sound of people on Doran Beach. You will be closing on the entrance to Tomales Bay, which has its own reputation as a great-white-shark park. When I make this trip, it's with a teammate I can rely on, and we leave a second vehicle at Nicks Cove, opposite Hog Island (Map 6).

From inside Bodega Harbor there are no great views of anything other than boats or mudflats. The flats are feeding ground for huge numbers and many species of shorebirds. The deep water is fishing territory for three species of loons, five different grebes, three types of tern, brown and white pelicans, three species of herons, three varieties of cormorants, and up to a dozen species of diving ducks. Some of these families of birds come and go with the seasons; some stay year round. In the spring, the black geese arrive in large numbers. These are small brant geese, not much bigger than a mallard, that feed almost exclusively on eel grass. They don't honk like other wild geese when they arrive, but mutter their background music with a low, growling sound. The word "brant" describes their true coloring from the Latin word brantus, *which is defined as "burnt black" or "black with a charred look." They are a wonderful sight to watch as they fly in from the sea, and when they've settled on the water you can observe that each one has a delicate white pendant either side of its black neck.*

Imagine you are kayaking with me in the harbor in April and we've worked our way up to the north end in the deep water. The tide is low, and we have no difficulty approaching shorebirds in our kayaks; unlike waterfowl, they simply don't rate kayaks as a threat. On the flats, we notice some little black 'pipers that are unlike all the others, which, whatever their size, from the long-billed curlew down to the least sandpiper, are brown or gray on their backs. It's a flock of black turnstones at the water's edge, querulously chattering and constantly on the move, industriously turning shells and other small objects over with their beaks. Their beaks are specially designed for this task.

Suddenly, the turnstones burst into flight, wheeling in a scything arc around us, so that they become vividly striped and patterned in black and white. They land close to us, and now they are black again. Like the brant geese, black and white in flight, the turnstones are predominantly black when they land. These turnstones and the geese are fueling up for the flight they are about to make, far away to the north. They both breed in the high latitudes from the Arctic coast of Alaska, right across to Baffin Island. What goes round and round in my head as I think of their long, upcoming flight are Walt Whitman's words, "All islands to which birds wing their way, I wing my way myself."

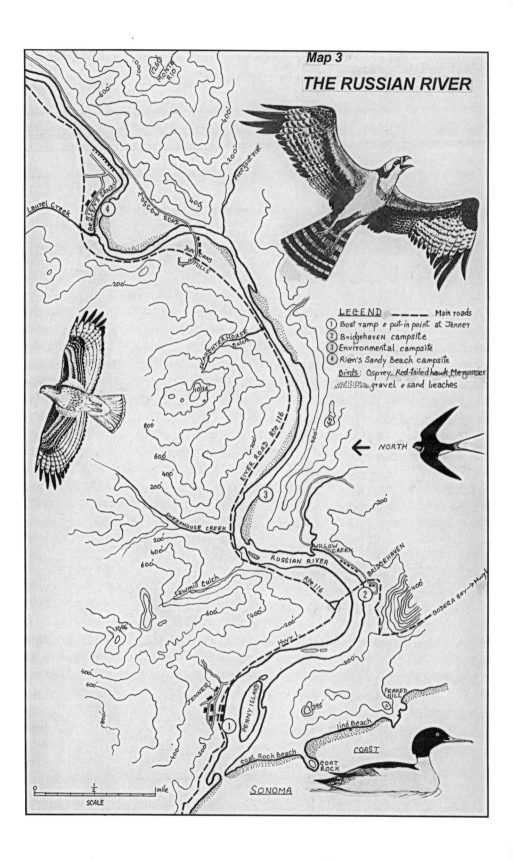

Map 3

THE RUSSIAN RIVER

LEGEND ――――― Main roads
① Boat ramp & put-in point at Jenner
② Bridgehaven campsite
③ Environmental campsite
④ Rien's Sandy Beach campsite
Birds: Osprey, Red-tailed hawk, Merganser
gravel & sand beaches

NORTH

MONTE RIO

1260'

600'

400'

200'

FREZOUT FLAT

Laurel Creek

RIEN'S SANDY

MOSCOW ROAD

④

600'

400'

200'

DUNCANS MILLS

SLAUGHTERHOUSE GULCH

1036'

800'

600'

400'

200'

RIVER ROAD Rte 116

③

651'

400'

200'

SHEEPHOUSE CREEK

200'

400'

600'

WILLOW CREEK

RUSSIAN RIVER

BRIDGEHAVEN

BODEGA BAY → Hwy 1

Sawmill Gulch

Rte 116

②

400'

1096'

600'

400'

200'

Hwy 1

200'

PEAKED HILL

JENNER

PENNY ISLAND

①

395'

lind Beach

COAST

Goat Rock Beach

GOAT ROCK

400'

600'

800'

200'

SONOMA

0   ¼   ½   1 mile
SCALE

TRIP 3 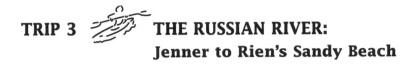 THE RUSSIAN RIVER:
Jenner to Rien's Sandy Beach

Type	Length	Map
Moderate day	13.5 miles RT to Rien's Sandy Beach	3
Easy overnight	13.5 miles RT to Rien's Sandy Beach	3
Easy overnight	5.5 miles RT to Environmental Campsite	3

Summary and Highlights

Suitable for canoe or kayak, this trip covers the Russian River Estuary, where it enters the Pacific Ocean below Jenner to Rien's Sandy Beach, 6.75 miles upstream. Jenner is only 8 miles south of Fort Ross, which was the stronghold of the Russian American Fur Company. Seal and otter hunting supported the Russians in this region until 1841. Now, the Russian River is a popular summer scene for swimming and boating, and noted for its winter steelhead fishing. There are two good commercial campsites and one "environmental" site available year round; all three have direct access to the water. Wildlife highlights include "fishhawks," ospreys, and the biggest of the "sawbills," American mergansers. I have seen coyotes and, once, a bobcat from my kayak.

How to Get There

Follow the route for Trips 1 and 2 to Bodega Bay, using the 76 gas station there as your zero mileage mark to continue north to Jenner on Route 1. After 2.1 miles, on your right you'll see two pretty ponds below you, and between them the flowing Salmon Creek. Continue north 6.4 miles. Then, driving steeply downhill, you'll come to the elegant modern bridge over the Russian River at BRIDGEHAVEN. Just before the bridge on the left, across from a large Indian restaurant, The Sizzling Tandoor, a narrow paved lane leads downhill into the BRIDGEHAVEN CAMPSITE. This commercial campsite is a discreet sanctuary with its own little beach giving access to the Russian River, 1 mile upstream from the public access to the river in Jenner. Tom O'Bryan is the manager (707) 865-2473. I recommend it as a base if you want to stay one or two nights in the area. It costs $20/night for up to five people/site. The restrooms have flush toilets and hot showers.

Continuing over the bridge toward Jenner, 0.5 mile beyond the Indian restaurant, Route 1 intersects Route 116. Stay on Route 1, turning left at this junction. The Russian River is now on your left, and in 1.1 miles you'll see on your left a business sign: SEAGULL GIFTS & DELI. Behind this building is another sign at the entrance to a small parking lot which gives direct access to a public boat ramp. It reads: SONOMA COAST STATE BEACH—JENNER—VISITOR CENTER. This is your destination.

You are surrounded by every amenity you could need, all visible from the entrance to the boat ramp: JENNER INN & COTTAGES, a bed and breakfast inn which is both extremely comfortable and elegant (800) 372-2377. There are a grocery store, a gas station, a post office, an information center, and public toilets at the boat ramp. I have left my truck in the free parking lot at the boat ramp overnight (you take your chances). Perhaps offering a small fee to park at the gas station across the road would be safer.

Trip Description: Downstream

In the spring I put in at the Jenner boat ramp and went straight down to the ocean, 0.75 mile away, passing Penny Island on my left. At the river's mouth the narrow cut through the sand, letting the river flow into the sea, had been human-made with bulldozers. This is done to avoid flooding, after the winter storms have blocked the estuary with sand. I could detect no taste of salt in the outflowing water, and that was consistent with the great activi-

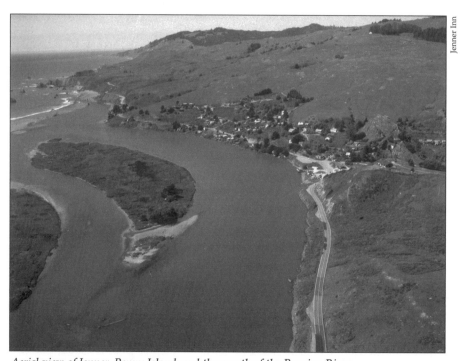

Aerial view of Jenner, Penny Island, and the mouth of the Russian River ty of small freshwater fish, six to nine inches long, that were leaping all over the place. These are steelhead trout on their first passage to the ocean—young fish that the locals call "smolts," as if they were salmon.

These one-year-olds have already, since December, run the gauntlet of dedicated recreational fly-fishers throughout the daylight hours. They've got by these hazardous hunters, who stand thigh-deep in the water waving their wands, all the way from the birthing grounds above Guerneville. Those that were caught were thrown back anyway. But the ospreys, cormorants, and mergansers don't release them. Down by the river mouth, the smolts have one last hazard to get by. They must run the gauntlet of the pinnipeds and the sea ravens, the double-crested cormorants. These predators are waiting on both banks at the gate to the maturation phase in the steelheads' life cycle.

On the left bank, looking seaward, are the "feather-footed" carnivores that prefer the aquatic life, the harbor seals. Like all harbor seals they are nervous when out of water. It could be they are genetically prepped to remember the Russian fur traders who used to hunt them on this river. Even as they lounge luxuriously on their side of the cut, they can become easily panic-stricken. On the other bank, separated from the seals by only 20 yards, are the insatiable sea ravens. They, too, are enjoying discretionary time at the outflow to the sea because the fishing is so easy here.

It's a federal offense to harass seals, and you must take care to avoid them when they've hauled out. All this sun-bathing they seem to enjoy is vital maintenance, a source of warmth and complete relaxation while their blood is reoxygenated for the long periods they spend under water. They sunbathe for their survival. So do the diving cormorants; after a fishing spell, their heraldic hanging out, with wings widespread, is to prevent their feathers from becoming waterlogged.

Trip Description: Upstream

Returning from the narrow rivermouth toward Jenner, you have the option of paddling the 0.5-mile passage between Penny Island and the south bank of the river. This channel is narrower than the way you went down to the sea and the island will block any sighting of Jenner as you head upstream.

A mile up from the ocean, the river will curve to the right, and you'll find two substantial gravel-bar islands on your left. The river is 200 yards wide at this point, so that you tend not to notice the changes in direction, but it now curves east and the Bridgehaven Bridge is 0.5 mile ahead. You are 1.8 miles upstream from the river's mouth. On the right bank there is a small beach, almost under the bridge, which is the put-in point from the Bridgehaven Campsite. Willow Creek enters the river 0.5 mile after the bridge, again on your right. It is only navigable a short distance on a high tide, but it has a marsh, out of sight from the river, that is a designated nature reserve.

The river curves north over the next mile, and a very shallow area is on your left. These shallows have some major tree trunks permanently embedded in them, and on these trunks you are likely to find seals, lying like large slugs. Then the river narrows abruptly where a point of land juts into it from your left, and on this promontory you'll recognize the foundation remains of a bridge. When you pass through the narrow section there will be a bay to your left. The river turns 90 degrees to the right and then keeps curving right, east, until it's heading southeast.

Paddling 0.5 mile from the promontory down this reach, you'll find the right bank is heavily wooded with tall firs and deciduous trees. There may now be ospreys calling and flying overhead. You'll see a long gravel shoal ahead to your left, but you should be watching the right bank closely because the best campsite on the river is close at hand. It's a small grassy plateau that comes right up to the water's edge and has a drop-off bank in front of it. It is 1.75 miles above Bridgehaven, and it's in the jurisdiction of the Sonoma Park Ranger Station on Route 1 at Salmon Creek (707) 875-2603. "First come, first served, year round," is the ruling I got when visiting the ranger station.

This site goes by the unofficial name of the "Environmental Campsite," and it is a precious site indeed. If you are in residence, anyone can see, from the water, that the place is taken, and there is no marked approach to the site from the nearest road. There is ample space for a small group of no more than six people, and kayaks can easily be hauled clear of the water—which they should be at night! A large fire pit and a weatherproof wood cabinet with matches and kindling wood are provided. (It's the responsibility of each person using this site to restock the kindling and make sure there are matches.)

Leaving the Environmental Campsite behind, your next available year-round site is a commercial one 3 miles farther upstream on the left bank. It is not named on the topo map, but you'll have no difficulty recognizing it when you get to it. The next 2 miles of the river run east in a nearly straight line, then the river turns north at the beginning of a large loop. As it begins to head north there are long, fine gravel bars on your left, where you pass under the Moscow Road Bridge. Its name is a further reminder of the past presence of the Russian hunters. If you need to, you can haul out on the left bank and walk 0.25 mile into Duncans Mills, where there are shops; otherwise, head north into the loop.

All the gravel bars on the river are within the jurisdiction of the Sonoma Parks system and may be used by boaters to haul out, but they may not be used for overnight camping. If you do use them, throughout the spring and early summer you'll be walking in the nesting grounds of killdeer plovers and spotted sandpipers. Both these birds lay four eggs in a scrape, or within a few tussocks of grass on open ground, and they rely for protection on the cryptic coloring of their eggs blending with the gravel. In the months of April,

May, and June, tread warily if you see these birds running around you. They call vigorously and run close ahead of you, hoping to draw you away from their nests.

Your loop of river is about to head east again with a major gravel bar to your right, but before it does, at the northernmost part of the loop, there is a large creek, Laurel Creek, entering the river from your left. At first sight, it looks navigable, but it isn't unless you get to it before the release of the spring floodwater at the mouth of the river, in other words, some time before or just into April.

Now, for the first time since you saw the ocean beach at the river's mouth, you'll be seeing clean yellow sand on the beaches ahead of you to your left. You have reached Rien's Sandy Beach, 6 miles above your put in at Jenner. Here, you can haul out, rest up, and return, or stay overnight at the campsite.

The owner claims that Rien's Sandy Beach is the only sand beach available as a campsite on the whole Russian River. It's open year-round for trailers, campers, and tenters. All the sites have drinking water and picnic tables; there are good bathrooms and hot showers. I recommend it because it's clean, well managed, and well situated on the river. This campsite has had an active osprey's nest, high in a fir tree in the middle of camp, for many years.

The manager at Rien's Sandy Beach is Alexis Alexander (707) 865-2102, and she is very helpful to boaters coming off the river. The cost is $17 for two people/site; add $2/additional person. You can almost certainly camp here without reservations during the months of October through April, though it seems wise to call ahead. In the summer season, you will have to make advance reservations.

Other Options

Instead of starting this Russian River trip at Jenner, you can start from Rien's Sandy Beach and head down to the ocean. You could also paddle 3 miles upstream to Monte Rio, or 6 miles to Guernewood Park, but be aware that these are heavily crowded areas in the summer months. If you want to start at Rien's Sandy Beach, your road route to the campsite/beach is as follows: cross the Russian River at Bridgehaven on Route 1; turn right (north) at the junction with Route 116; drive 4 miles to Duncans Mills, where there are shops to your right; go another 1.5 miles on Route 116 and turn right onto Laurel Dell; drive 0.25 mile down Laurel Dell and turn right onto Sylvan Way. It will take you right into Rien's Sandy Camp and up to the office.

Imagine you are starting your journey from Jenner with me, now. We have the prevailing northwest wind behind us; as we head upstream, Penny Island, which is half a mile long, is to our right. From a sand spit at its east end we enjoy the sight and the raucous sound of a whole colony of big, bold Caspian terns. Those on the spit stand tidily on short legs, all facing upstream, while those in the air wheel in circles, pause in the air for target calculations, and hit the water solidly as they dive for fingerlings. And all the time, these Caspians scream and scream. They are gull-sized with a cleft tail, without the streamers that most terns have; and their powerful, vermilion beaks would make a great lipstick ad.

By the time we reach the bridge at Bridgehaven we're already seeing and hearing fishhawks. Their cries attract us long before we see our first one. These are ospreys whose high, plaintive, repetitive, and tuneless mono-piping call is nonetheless an urgent sound that carries far.

A handsome drake American merganser is swimming ahead of us, quite unafraid as we catch up to him. He has his tail widespread and cocked up high above the water; clearly he's using it as a sail, allowing the strong breeze to push him along. It's a most amusing trick to watch, but he's watching us over his shoulder, too; so though we seem to be sharing common ground, we steer wide enough away from him not to spoil his sailing initiative.

After Bridgehaven, the river is wide. Willow Creek enters the river on the right, and on the left bank there are shallows and grassy slopes leading onto open pasture. Many cows are grazing placidly over there, and at the water's edge we see a small flock of heavy, brown-and-white Emden geese with one much smaller, trim, white goose in their company. We paddle across to check them out: six great big, overweight farmyard honkers sharing the pastoral life with a stranger.

These geese have lived on this part of the river for years, quite wild. Two winters ago they were joined by a snow-white Ross goose—one of those Arctic breeding geese that fall out of their own flock, from either sickness or a gunshot wound, while wintering in the south. This one must have seen or heard the feral geese as it flew over the river, and when it came down to land it found itself safe with foster-friends on the cow-grazed meadows alongside the Russian River. They are all cautious, but we can see that the Ross goose is the shyest as we give them a wide berth.

We keep on meeting cormorants much smaller than those down at the estuary. As they come by in pairs we see that one in each pair has a beautiful white rump and flank patch singing it out as the male; they are pelagic cormorants. Soon fish-

hawks are everywhere, as the open pasture on the banks gives way to woods, and we see tall, old trees up ahead. We are entering well-known osprey breeding territory.

We made a late start today; in an hour's time it will be dusk and we need a good campsite. The best on the river designated for public use is up ahead of us now, on the right bank. It's not all that obvious, but it's the first time since we've had woods instead of open ground flanking us that a plateau of grass has appeared. So we go ashore to check it out and find it's ideal for a small group.

It's very peaceful. Tree swallows and barn swallows are hawking for insects, winding loop-ribbons over the water. A great blue heron is standing, patiently poised to make its next kill on the opposite side of the river. Steelhead and shad, a herring-like salt-water fish that also breeds in this river, are being almost herded, it seems, as ospreys line themselves up to dive. They are working much like collies cutting out sheep. At dusk a great-horned owl sounds its hollow "hoot." The night crow, Nycticorax, *sees us as it flies by and calls out crossly, "woc woc." And, after we've eaten together, each one of us withdraws into our own space to watch the night overtake the day. Here we'll sleep and spend the night undisturbed, after lying awake a while interpreting the night's sounds. I only wish I might hear the dog-like barks of a spotted owl.*

The spotted owl may no longer breed here, perhaps because there aren't enough woodrats to support it. It takes two colonies of woodrats in a pair of spotted owls' territory for them to be able to raise their young. So I think about the little steelheads that made it out to sea today. Those that aren't eaten by fish bigger than themselves will be out there for the next two years before they return to this river to breed. A few will make the trip back upstream and out to sea again, two or three times. And some will grow to weigh as much as 20 pounds. That's why all those fly-fishers, patient as that heron across the river there, will be back next December. And the next.

—•—⚓—•—

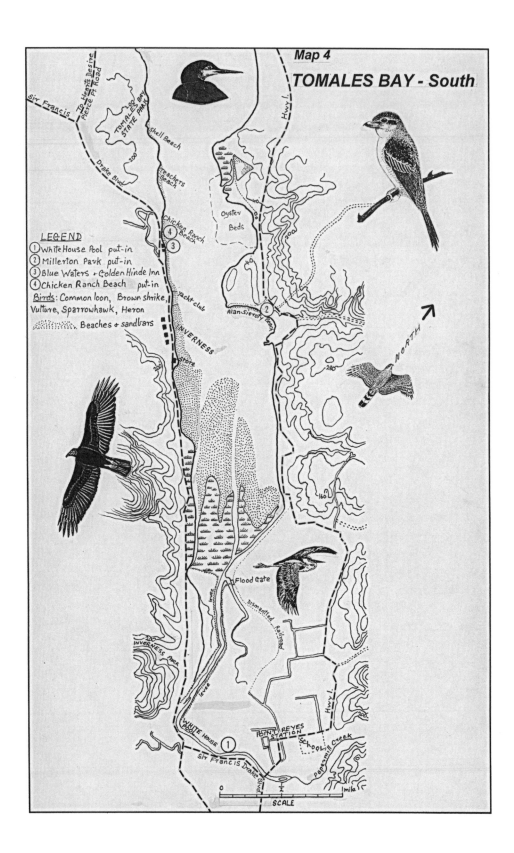

Map 4

TOMALES BAY - South

Sir Francis

To Heart's Desire
Pierce Pt. Road

TOMALES BAY STATE PARK

Drake Blvd.

Shell Beach

Treachers Beach

Oyster Beds

Hwy. 1

LEGEND
① White House Pool put-in
② Millerton Park put-in
③ Blue Waters + Golden Hinde Inn
④ Chicken Ranch Beach put-in
Birds: Common loon, Brown shrike,
Vulture, Sparrowhawk, Heron
Beaches + sandbars

Chicken Ranch Beach

④
③

Yacht club

Alan Sieroty Beach

②

INVERNESS

NORTH

store

Flood Gate

Dismantled Railroad

INVERNESS PARK

Hwy. 1

WHITE HOUSE

POINT REYES STATION

School Creek

Papermill Creek

Sir Francis Drake Blvd.

①

0   1 mile
SCALE

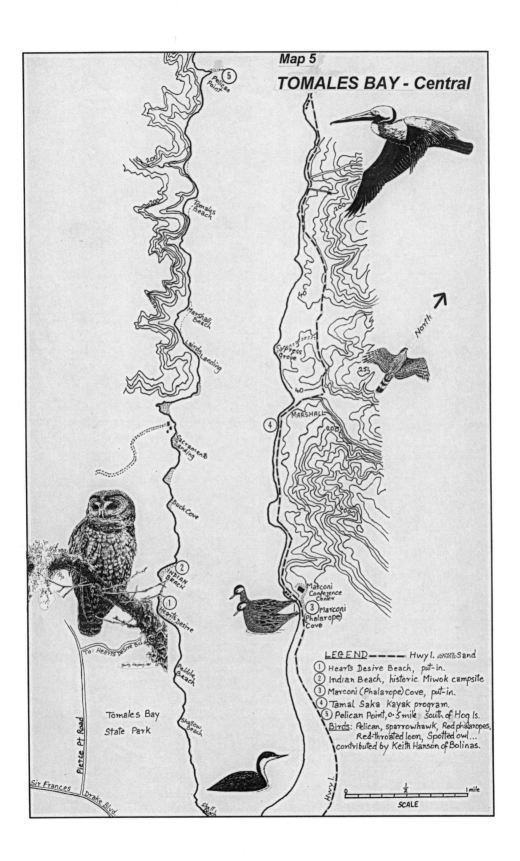

Map 5

TOMALES BAY - Central

Pelican Point ⑤

200

Tomales Beach

200

North ↗

Marshall Beach

Laird's Landing

Cypress Grove

251

40

MARSHALL

Sacramento Landing

④

200

Duck Cove

② INDIAN BEACH

① Hearts Desire

To: Hearts Desire Bd.

Marconi Conference Center

③ Marconi (Phalarope) Cove

Pebble Beach

Tomales Bay State Park

shallow beach

LEGEND ---- Hwy 1. ≈≈≈Sand

① Hearts Desire Beach, put-in.
② Indian Beach, historic Miwok campsite
③ Marconi (Phalarope) Cove, put-in.
④ Tamal Saka Kayak program.
⑤ Pelican Point, 0.5 mile south of Hog Is.
Birds: Pelican, sparrowhawk, Red phalaropes, Red-throated loon, Spotted owl... contributed by Keith Hanson of Bolinas.

Pierce Pt. Road

Sir Frances Drake Blvd.

shell beach

Hwy 1.

0   ½   1 mile

SCALE

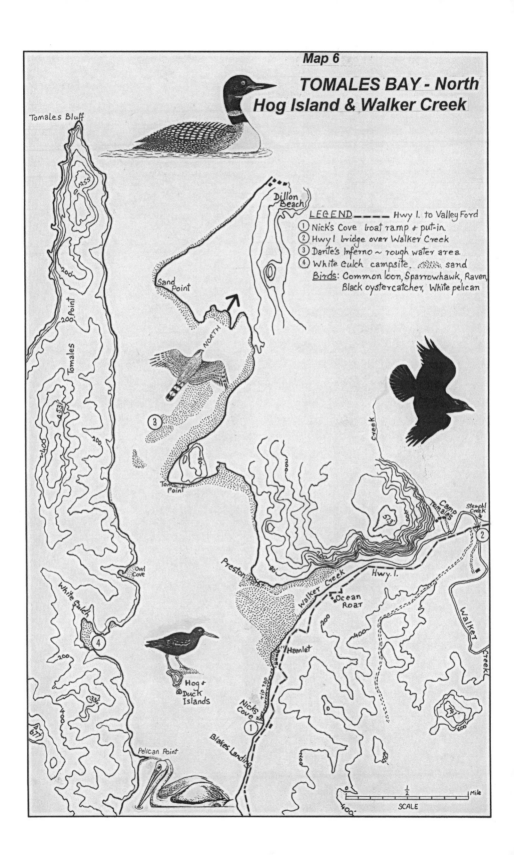

Map 6

TOMALES BAY - North
Hog Island & Walker Creek

Tomales Bluff

Dillon Beach

LEGEND ━ ━ ━ ━ Hwy I. to Valley Ford
1 Nick's Cove boat ramp & put-in
2 Hwy I bridge over Walker Creek
3 Dante's Inferno ~ rough water area
4 White Gulch campsite. ⣿⣿⣿ sand
Birds: Common loon, Sparrowhawk, Raven, Black oystercatcher, White pelican

Sand Point

NORTH

Tomales Point

3

Tomales Point

Owl Cove

White Gulch

4

Creek

Camp Tomales

Stemphl Creek

2

Preston Point

Walker Creek

Hwy. I.

Walker Creek

Ocean Roar

Hamlet

Hog & Duck Islands

Nicks Cove Rd.

1

Blakes Landing

Pelican Point

0   ½   Mile
SCALE

Chapter 4

Tomales Bay

TRIP 4 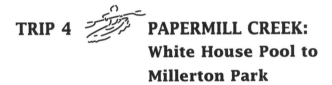 PAPERMILL CREEK: White House Pool to Millerton Park

Type	Length	Map
Moderate half day	7.5 miles RT to Millerton Park	4
Easy half day	4 miles RT to delta	4

Summary and Highlights

This tidal creek is shallow, but navigable, and, for 2 miles, very safe for newcomers to kayaking and canoeing. Putting in at White House Pool in Papermill Creek, paddling to the creek's delta—possibly as far as Millerton Park—and returning, is a half-day trip. It could become a long half day if you go this far, and you'll need a day with a good high tide to do it because Millerton Point and Millerton Park are 3.75 miles from White House Pool. The creek fans out into a delta as it enters Tomales Bay. Once you are in the bay, the wind will usually be fresh and coming right at you, unless you are on the water early. The birdlife in the delta area is outstanding because the nutrients for shorebirds, terns, cormorants and white pelicans are most abundant here.

One of the rarest birds to be seen in North America, the Siberian red-tailed shrike, inhabited the huge Himalaya blackberry bushes at White House Pool for several months in 1987. Virginia rails, cattle egrets, sandhill cranes, and emperor geese are among the rarities that I've seen in the reeds and on the marshes surrounding this creek.

Special Advice

Paddling this route calls for close attention to the tide book. You have two hours either side of high tide (more if the tides are higher than average) in which to go out on the rising tide as far as Millerton Park (3.75 miles), and get back before the tide has fallen. (Always explore shallow routes on a rising tide, not on a falling tide, so that you can withdraw without getting stuck in the mud.)

How to Get There

Coming from the east: use the Richmond-San Rafael Bridge; pass under Route 101 at Larkspur; and drive west on Sir Francis Drake Blvd. Coming from the south on Route 101, take SIR FRANCES DRAKE BLVD. EXIT at Larkspur, and turn left onto the same route. It is 23 miles from Larkspur to White House Pool, all of it on Sir Frances Drake Blvd.

Turn left at the T-junction lights in San Anselmo, 3.6 miles from the Route 1 exit. At 13 miles you enter SAMUEL P. TAYLOR STATE PARK. Where Sir Francis Drake Blvd. meets Shoreline Highway Route 1 in Olema (20.3 miles), turn right for Point Reyes Station. At 22.2 miles, immediately before the bridge leading into Point Reyes Station, turn left off Route 1. In 0.7 mile from the turnoff, on your right is a road into a parking lot. The sign, WHITE HOUSE POOL—PUBLIC ACCESS, is not visible until you turn into the access. This is your put-in point for Papermill Creek. There is a toilet and free parking space, open from 4 A.M. to 9 P.M.

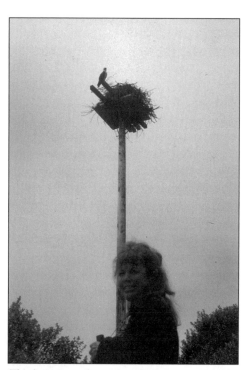

This human-made nesting site for ospreys at Millerton Park is occupied every spring

Trip Description

There is grass and a solid park bench right where you'll slide your boat down the bank into the water. The water is always calm here, but tidal and slow moving. You should note which way it's

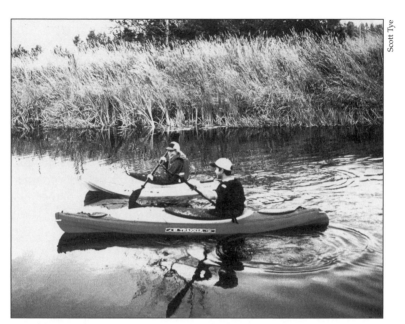

Small kayaks like these Trakkers are ideal for first-timers on Papermill Creek

flowing. You will be heading left, west, when you get on the water, and if the water's going with you, then you are on a falling tide. Be aware of the times of high and low tide and your own time frame for returning.

You'll head west for 0.2 mile and then turn north on a mile-long reach. Willow trees and blackberry bushes are on both banks, and between you and them are tall, green rushes behind which the Virginia rail lives its secretive life. The trees, the briars, and the rushes are filled with small passerines—birds that perch, and most of which are inclined to sing. Blackbirds, thrushes, sparrows, warblers, and marsh wrens will applaud and scold you all the way as you pass through their territory.

After this first mile, a long, narrow island is detached from the right bank by only a few yards, just enough to make a navigable channel (not shown on the map). It's best passed on the left if you want to maintain your view over the marshes. After the island, the creek gets wider and will bend to the west a little and curve back to the north for another mile. The banks of the creek have only pickleweed and grasses behind them now, so that white egrets and great-blue herons have replaced the singing birds. Look out for white-tailed kites and northern harriers because they thrive by flying low over the marshes here. They are called the "searchers" rather than "attackers" among the birds of prey; they quarter the ground in a meandering, tireless quest for mice.

After these two miles of paddling you are in the shallow delta that fans out into the bay. It's an impressive sight. It is also one of the two areas in Tomales

Bay that cannot be used all the time. North of Millerton Point, the bay is navigable at any state of the tide, except for the delta of Walker Creek, 9 miles farther north, which is another feeding ground for shorebirds. In the summer, if you're lucky, you may meet up with the local flock of white pelicans, standing in the shallows and on the sandy mudbars to your left or right. There will be a few dead trees, lying stranded in the delta mud, convenient as perches for cormorants. And by now you'll be well aware of the breeze coming at you from the north. This is the easy, half-day trip destination, and point of return.

The bay beyond the delta is now almost a mile wide. You'll see Millerton Point jutting from the right shore, 1.75 miles ahead of you. This point is a half-mile long and forms its own bay where it juts out from the mainland. Millerton Park is tucked into the corner from which this point starts, and, viewed from your kayak, there is nothing by which to identify it. However, as you come out of the delta, a long line of stakes, the remains of oyster racks, leads you toward Millerton Park. Stay close to these and follow them, always conscious that you want to close on the land ahead well to the right of the western tip of Millerton Point.

As you approach Millerton Park, one detail begins to stand out above other features on the shoreline ahead. It is a lone telegraph pole on the skyline, directly above Millerton Park. On the top of this pole is a human-made platform with an ospreys' nest of large sticks built on it. It is a great landmark, year round, and has been occupied ever since it was set up for the ospreys. Aim for the ospreys' nest and you will home in on the park.

⊷ ≋◊≋ ⊶

It's early April as I put in at White House Pool on a rising tide, knowing it will let me get back. My trip starts in an idyllic, sheltered spot and takes me north, into Tomales Bay. But, by the time I get into the bay, the wind gets up.

As I push off from the bank, there is a fox sparrow ten feet away, hopping and kicking back the soil, just as a towhee does. Its breast is spotted like a thrush's and it's much bigger than any other sparrow. On both banks, either side of me, red-winged blackbirds flash their epaulets and sing their heads off from the tops of tall rushes. "Conk-ka-reee," they call, and pause to see what effect that has. Farther on, a black phoebe is demonstrating its fly-catching skill over the water. Then a female kingfisher, recognizable by its rust-red vest, rattles off its call—like a telephone ringing—as it flies ahead of me to find another perch.

My kayak's bow is slicing through the water as I cruise along, setting up two, little bow waves 35 degrees off my line of travel. I focus on these ripples of water, one coming from each side of my bow, and spear them with my paddle, as close to the bow as my reach allows. This is the exact point at which the blade should enter the water. My upper body rotates slightly with each stroke, and I pull my hands toward my hips on almost straightened arms. I don't think of putting water behind me with each stroke: I pull the boat up to the blade. It's a subtle mental aid, akin to thinking of the glass half-full rather than half-empty. All these things I do automatically, but whenever I kayak I also look in on what I'm doing—a sort of quality control.

I glide by a pair of western grebes that barely take the trouble to swim around me; they are taking a grebe-nap, with their heads nestled on their backs. And now I see a female American merganser ahead of me. She flies off with a clatter of wings slapping the water, and I know her partner is somewhere up ahead. I know it because the two pairs of these large diving ducks that breed here are old friends of mine. Within the next mile I anticipate seeing another species of merganser, the red-breasted. It's unusual for these two "sawbills" to be seen so close together. Mergansers are called "sawbills" because of their long, pincer-like beaks, which have clearly-visible, serrated edges, the better to grip their slippery prey.

Up ahead I see two unlikely looking birds standing up to their thighs in shallow water. They aren't white, and don't stand like egrets; they aren't black, but do have a vulturine posture. They are big, brown-backed birds, quite still; and now one of them makes a move so that I see it has a white front. They are ospreys. I think of these fishhawks diving dramatically from the sky for their food, not hanging out like cormorants and mergansers. But there they are, and once I saw one carrying a watervole, instead of a fish, away from this area.

I'm working quite hard now in my cormorant-black Arluk II because the wind is getting up. I hear a spotted sandpiper's weeping call to my left, and there it is, flying along the muddy edge of the water. Its wings go "sputter-glide, sputter-glide," like a motor that keeps cutting out. As I get to the delta, a small gray loon surfaces just in front of me, leaving most of its body submerged. As soon as it sees me it slides under the surface, so I stop paddling to let it get ahead of me. Now it pops up with all its body in view, holding its head at the angle typical of a red-throated loon, as if it's looking for something over the horizon.

In spite of the wind I strike out boldly for Millerton Park. Little white caps are dancing all around me on pummeling waves. Many red-breasted mergansers are scattering ahead of me; they don't want to fly in this wind. A Caspian tern dives right in front of me and carries off a prize-winning, five-inch fish. The fish squiggles like mad and almost gets away as the tern tries to improve its grip. But the big, gull-like tern has it, and I learn that it can carry a big fish and scream at the same time.

I'm out in the bay and the waves are forcing me to pay attention to my survival. I aim for Millerton Point rather than the park so that I can paddle into the eye of the wind and meet the waves head on. Before long I'm near the bench that's used by hikers who walk out to the point, and I turn about. I'm glad I didn't come out in my Navarro today; a canoe would simply be thrown back by the wind in these conditions.

Normally, what I've just done makes a leisurely, half-day trip. Today it takes me an hour and fifteen minutes to reach Millerton Point, but I rip back with the wind dead astern, surfing a galloping, following sea. I'm riding endless two-foot waves. They are perfectly shaped and evenly spaced, close together, about ten yards apart. I chase, catch, and ride each wave ahead of me as I race home. It's just like running down an endless escalator that's already going my way. In 35 minutes I'm at my truck.

TRIP 5 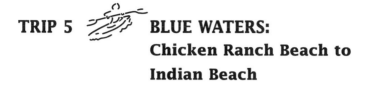 BLUE WATERS:
Chicken Ranch Beach to
Indian Beach

Type	Length	Map
Easy half day	5.5 miles RT to Indian Beach	4 & 5

Summary and Highlights

The trip described here is a guided tour by the Blue Waters Sea Kayaking Program, out of Inverness. Putting in from Chicken Ranch Beach, our destination highlight is a potluck lunch and seminar on the ancient Coastal Miwok midden at Indian Beach. After a 2.75-mile paddle, Tomales Bay State Park Ranger, Carlos Porrata, will join us and share his knowledge of the bay's human and natural history. Overlooking the ancient midden is the forest from which the Miwok gathered much of their food, and where the endangered spotted owl still breeds. I highly recommend you take the Blue Waters trip because of Ranger Porrata's fascinating and entertaining guided tour of Indian Beach.

Blue Waters (415) 669-7835 operates from the Golden Hinde Inn (415) 669-1389, at Inverness. Call Blue Waters to find out when this summer-season trip is scheduled. Blue Waters offers a variety of on-water safety classes and kayak-touring experiences from the more-sheltered side of the bay. Blue Waters' parking lot and office are immediately behind the inn's reception office, and they have bathroom facilities. The owner is Kate McClain.

How to Get There

Follow the route for Trip 4 to White House Pool and continue north on Sir Francis Drake Blvd., toward Inverness. The road follows Papermill Creek, which is on your right. If you are coming from the south, on Shoreline Highway Route 1, drive 15.4 miles from Highway 101 through Stinson Beach to Olema. From Olema, follow the route for Trip 4.

At 0.5 mile after White House Pool, a sign on your right reads: INVERNESS PARK. 2.5 miles after this sign you reach the small town of Inverness. The Inverness Store and a gas station are side by side on your right; both are open seven days a week, year round. There's an excellent bakery across the road from the store.

One mile north of Inverness, the Golden Hinde Inn is on your right. It is a comfortable, inexpensive motel, ideally situated for a kayaking weekend on the bay. You can put in at all tides from the inn's mini-beach, without charge if you are a guest. There is a $10 parking and launching fee if you are not. Only 30 yards past the entrance to the inn's parking lot, a narrow, paved driveway leads into the parking lot for the Blue Waters outfit. Their office is in the same block as the inn reservations office, and should be entered from the kayaking/parking lot.

For free access to the bay in this immediate area, not on either the Golden Hinde's or the Blue Waters' property, drive 100 yards north of the Blue Waters' entrance to gain access to Chicken Ranch Beach. There is a shoulder for road-side parking on your right, with a clearly defined gap in the hedge for foot traffic down to the water's edge. There is a public toilet at this gap. One bonus for this public put-in point is that it has no opening or closing time.

Trip Description

You can, of course, head out for any site you choose in the bay from the three, adjacent put-in points described here. But, if you are renting a boat from Blue Waters, they will quiz your previous kayaking experience before deciding what sort of craft to rent to you. This is a necessary safety factor and a responsibility they take on. The trip is not very far, only about 3 miles, and what you see along the way and when you get there, is always pleasurable.

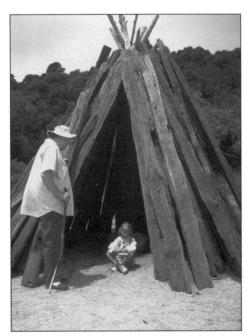

A child and her grandmother enjoy a kotca *replica on Indian Beach*

But what you can learn from Ranger Carlos Porrata is the focal point of the day.

Carlos will direct your eyes, extend your vision, and share his passion for Tomales Bay. He has a masters degree in education and has been a Tomales Bay State Park Ranger for 20 years. His interest in Coastal Miwok natural history and social culture crystalizes on Indian Beach. It is here that he demonstrates an Environmental Living Program, giving work-shops for school teachers who, in turn, bring children to Indian Beach for an environmental-living, overnight experience.

On this Blue Waters trip, you put in from Chicken Ranch Beach in the corner adjacent to the Golden Hinde Inn. The wind will

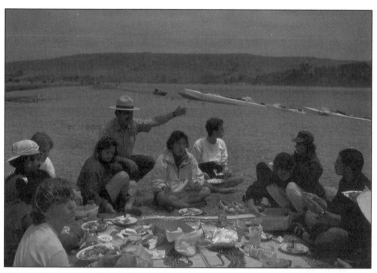

Ranger Porrata explains Miwok social history over a potluck lunch

probably be coming from the northwest. Staying close to the west shore for shelter, in 0.5 mile you'll be opposite Teachers Beach, and in another 0.3 mile you'll come to a series of tall, red-and-white marker buoys, placed along your route. Leave them on your left; they mark a designated swimming area off Shell Beach. At 1.5 miles you'll pass Shallow Beach, which is in a pleasantly sheltered cove. You are off Pebble Beach at 2 miles. Much of this reach of the west shore is rocky, and it has cliffs on a small scale. Where you are paddling the water looks deep, but there are submerged rocks close to the surface. So, don't paddle too close to shore.

Looking up at the cliffs you'll see large weeping patches of orange-red, and this vivid coloring indicates concentrations of iron ore in the rock. Above the edge of the cliffs, you'll see pine trees that don't stand as tall as you would expect for their girth. They have a rumpled look. These are Bishop pines, indigenous to the area; and there are other trees up there, including three species of oak, all of which produce acorns that feed jays and woodpeckers. They used to feed the original inhabitants of the area, too—the Coastal Miwok.

At 2.5 miles, you can see Indian Beach dead ahead, but before you get to it there's another beach, hiding in a corner of the shoreline, which is suddenly in sight. It is the most popular beach in the bay, Hearts Desire. You can see now that you could walk along this beach to get to Indian Beach. In fact there is an "Indian Nature Trail," which you can't see from the water, developed by Carlos Porrata. It starts behind the washrooms at Hearts Desire and leads you, cross-country, to Indian Beach. This short hike is designed to show you the plants, shrubs, and trees that helped sustain the indigenous people of Tomales Bay who lived here an estimated 3,500 years ago.

On this lovely day in early July we sit around a big blanket, with all the good things people can think of to bring to a potluck lunch. While we eat, Carlos talks about the human history and the natural history of Tomales Bay. He reminds us that "the People" is the right term for any race of first inhabitants in any place. The word "Indian" is a complete misnomer given the native people by Europeans who reached this continent and thought they had hit India.

We enjoy our lunch while sitting on a midden, with three kotcas *(shelters) alongside us. A midden is one of those obvious features that we can walk right over on a beach without knowing it, if we don't have Carlos Porrata's educated eye. It is a slightly elevated plateau in the sand. The color is quite different from the sand surrounding it; a dirty white shade compared with the yellowish shade of sand. When this was pointed out, it was easy to see that a midden is a specific place, in an empty space. Tribal members had lived on this beach and, year after year, cracked oysters and other shellfish, cooked and ate them sitting in this tennis-court-sized spot.*

Eventually, the surface of this area, the epicenter of a communal life, was completely changed. No longer a sand surface, it became an elevated raised platform surface of crushed shells and charcoal, as fine as the sand. But by digging into a midden, a way of living is revealed. Carbon dating of materials from the midden proves that people were cooking here more than 1,000 years ago. The three kotcas, *the Miwok shelters on Indian Beach, are made from long slabs of tree bark, stacked upright to form a tall cone. Carlos and his colleagues in the Park Service built these to replicate one of the styles of housing used by "the People" of Tomales Bay.*

Life for the Coastal Miwok living in Tomales Bay was good. Deer, fish, oysters, clams, crabs, berries, nuts, and fruit were abundant. The temperature was mild in winter, not too hot in summer, and fresh water flowed from every gulch around the bay. They even had soap with which to wash, using the bulb of the amole, or soap plant. And they had saka, *"the boat." Their water transport was made from tightly bound roles of tules and other reeds, lashed together to make a canoe-like vessel. They used it until it became waterlogged, and then they built more. On the east side of the bay, the kayak program, Tamal Saka, operating out of Marshall on Tomales Bay (415) 663-1743, has one of these Coastal Miwok* saka *as its logo. John Granatir, from this program, tells me that* Tamal saka *means "the boat of the bay."*

TRIP 6 HEARTS DESIRE BEACH TO HOG ISLAND

Type	Length	Map
Moderate day	10 miles RT to Hog Island	5 & 6

Summary and Highlights

Hearts Desire Beach is a park facility open from 8 A.M. to 8 P.M., with a $5 day/car fee. It is the most popular Tomales Bay beach in summer, with flush toilets and plenty of parking space. This is an active site, a family place for swimmers, boaters, and picnickers, with a designated swimming area. It's a safe place for children to play in small rubber dinghies and sit-on kayaks; and it's the best westshore, put-in point for kayakers because of its position, midway on the 15-mile length of the bay. Many kayak-touring programs start trips from here, to reach any of the wide variety of destinations in the bay. The day trips, using the tides and wind wisely, that you can make from this beach include going as far as Toms Point or into Walker Creek, with numerous other options. Hog Island, 5 miles toward the ocean, is a favorite day trip.

Special Advice

Kayakers must take their boats over to the far right side of the beach for their put in, and use the same area to land. Work your way up into the wind on your outgoing route and come home with the wind. The wind in this bay is far more forceful than the tidal movement, so head north toward the ocean and Bodega Bay. On windy days, stay along the sheltered, west shore. When landing at Hearts Desire, make sure your kayak is not pointing at anyone, especially children, at the water's edge. Small waves often take control of your kayak the last few yards from the beach, and you cannot stop its momentum or erratic direction once this happens.

How to Get There

Follow the route for Trip 5. From the Golden Hinde Inn, continue north on Sir Frances Drake Blvd. In 0.5 mile, as the road swings west and uphill, away from the bay, the Inverness Valley Inn will be on your left; and, 0.8 mile beyond it, on your right a sign greets you: POINT REYES NATIONAL SEASHORE. After another 0.3 mile there's a smaller sign on your right: TOMALES STATE PARK—MCCLURES BEACH, with an arrow indicating that you leave Sir Frances Drake Blvd. to get to it. While Hearts Desire Beach is not mentioned, McClures Beach is the sign you follow onto Pierce Pt. Road. This road takes you uphill and along a ridge, with forest on your right and a panoramic view to your left. In 1.2 miles, almost out of sight from the road, on your right, you come to the sign for HEARTS DESIRE BEACH. Turn right and go downhill 0.8 mile to the park office, where your parking fee is taken. (Off season you must leave $5 in the fee box and place the receipt in your car window. Vehicles in the parking lot are checked in winter months.) From the office there is still another 0.5 mile to drive downhill. Turn left to the parking lot, toilet, and beach.

Trip Description

Going north, toward the mouth of the bay, Hog Island and its small satellite, Duck Island (otherwise known as Piglet), wait to be explored. Indian Beach, 0.5 mile ahead, and Pelican Point, 4 miles away, stand out. From there, 0.75 mile farther, but in the middle of the bay, is your goal. Hog Island is in sight all the time as you paddle down the bay. If you try to camp on this island, the wind itself will be very hard to take and the noise of the wind in the trees is extreme. There are plenty of sand beaches, out of the wind, on the west shore of Tomales Bay for camping, and at this time (summer 1997), if there are no buildings or signs denying access, there is no restriction on their use. (Owing to the rapid growth of kayak touring, this situation may change soon. Check with the park ranger when you arrive at Hearts Desire, or call Tomales Bay State Park (415) 669-1140.)

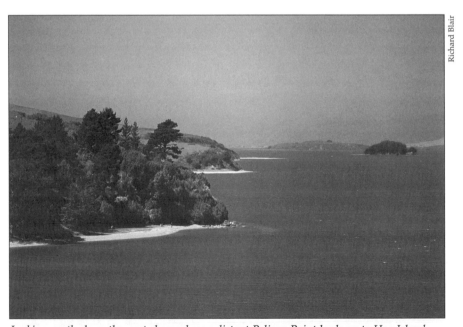

Looking north along the west shore where a distant Pelican Point leads on to Hog Island

Richard Blair

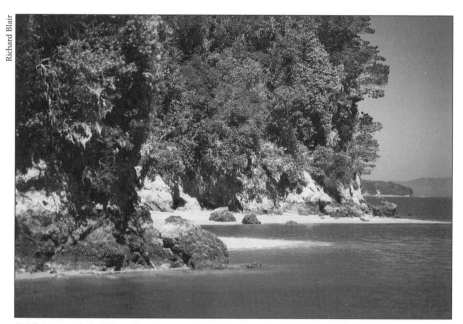

With its wooded cliffs and many coves, Tomales Bay's west shore is ideal for kayakers

Going further north: On the east shore, 1 mile north of Hog Island, you can head for Preston Point, explore the Walker Creek delta, and go 3.5 miles up the creek (but only on a flooding tide). The next point on the east shore is Toms Point, 1.5 miles beyond Hog Island. Finally, 3 miles beyond Hog Island, also on the east shore, there's Sand Point. This is the gateway to the bay, and it's as far as you should go unless you are experienced and equipped for ocean conditions.

When you reach Sand Point you'll experience a transition in the motion of the water. From the normal chop of any water exposed to wind, there will be added a slow, rocking motion that seems to have no direction. It's as though you are being moved around on a giant waterbed. This is caused by the ocean swells as they come into the bay through its opening and are met by shores that don't absorb them. They reflect them, "return to sender," so that the incoming and reflected swells meet. You experience an odd feeling that can cause motion sickness. For most people it's a signal to turn around and go back into the bay.

If you're an expert paddler and want an adrenaline shot, an area just west of Toms Point, about the size of a three-acre field, is one of the wildest pota-to patches, without any rocks involved, that you could wish to play in. Enter it only at your own risk. When it's cooking, it's perfectly obvious where it is because it looks like a cauldron of boiling water. It is generated at a certain period in the tide when currents clash over a sandbar that is always submerged. The sandbar has contours that encourage the disturbance. At the surface, the effect is impressive; and, if you venture into the turbulence, the effect will be like playing bumper cars with the waves that sprout out of nowhere and collide with each other and you. I call it Dante's Inferno. Don't go in there unless you have a really reliable combat roll in your escape kit. I've often played in it, but when I've gone in with a friend, the friend has always disappeared from my view. There is no way you can do anything except look after yourself; your friend can't help you, either.

Going south: Paddling south, and slightly east, from Hearts Desire Beach toward Papermill Creek and Point Reyes Station, there are no environmental camp sites; but there is the Golden Hinde Inn with its own marina and beach available if you intend staying there (see Trip 5). You can land at Chicken Ranch Beach near the Blue Waters kayaking operation. Everything south of Blue Waters is rather shallow, and you'll have to pay attention to your tide book before venturing any farther. But, well before low tide, you can land behind the Inverness Store (Map 4) and get supplies if needed.

Hearts Desire Beach offers the widest range of day trips on Tomales Bay. The fact that it is on the west shore gives you the best wind protection, most days of the year, but not always! The bird life is interesting year round, and at its best in the spring. The bay is quite famous for its varieties of jellyfish, and there are bat rays and harmless leopard sharks. There are always rumors of great whites in the bay, but in 15 years I've neither seen one, nor met anyone who has seen a great white shark inside Tomales Bay. But I'm not saying they aren't there. It's a good crabbing bay, and for this you need a license, just as you do for fishing. The best fish caught here are flounders, often around eight to twelve pounds. On weekdays you meet few other people, even in the summer, unless you land on one of the more popular bathing beaches, close to Inverness.

━━ ☙❦☙ ━━

On June 23, I've joined three friends at Hearts Desire Beach. By 10:30 a.m., the wind, coming directly from the north, is up. The wind normally blows straight up the bay from the west and today it's more northerly. This means there'll be protection from the west shore only if we're in one of the coves, or behind a point. While the cove at Heart's Desire is well sheltered, white caps are dancing downwind in the sunlight out in the big bay. The quality of the kayaks we're using today will be a major factor in our efforts to reach Hog Island. We are using particularly good boats: I'm in my black Arluk II; Paul is in the Seaward Cobra that Catherine Sliming used when we were "Shooting the Golden Gate;" and Martha and

Michael are in a new Necky boat, the Nootka. I think this fast double kayak is about the best kevlar-constructed craft of its kind.

My friends are not veteran kayakers; in fact, they're fairly new to it, but strong and willing. They have gone through wet-exit and reentry training. As soon as we leave the cove, it's obviously going to be an "adventure kayakers" day. Either that, or, like every group we see, we'll have to run for cover in the lee of the nearest wind-protected beach and stay there till it's time to go home.

We plow into the waves, working our way close inshore around the bluffs and into the bigger coves for well-earned breathers before going out again and continuing north into the bay. The secret is consistency. It's no good working hard and taking rests because we'll loose more yardage resting than we'll make when we're working. That, and keeping our bows constantly into the weather, will get us where we want to go.

Our goal is Hog Island, a benchmark feature in the bay, because my friends are keen to see the black oystercatchers that are breeding there. Our first 0.5 mile takes us past Indian Beach, where the Miwok shelters look to Paul like stacks of driftwood set up to make beach fires. We pass Duck Cove at 1 mile and Sacramento Landing at 1.5 miles, where the peacocks scream in response to my yodel. They never let me down. Then we turn into the large cove between Sacramento and Laird's landings and paddle across it, well out of the wind. There's a good term to describe a wind like today's, Down Under: it's called a "lazy wind." And that's because it doesn't bother to go around you.

Going into the big cove between the two landings pays off nicely when we see a male, pelagic cormorant, with its white flank patch identifying it, and a raft of "skunk heads" with brightly colored bills. These are surf scoters, an entirely male group of about 40 birds, with discretionary time because none are diving for food. They eat well here off shellfish and crabs. The white badges, on their foreheads and napes, contrast vividly with the rest of their blackness. And the wind-whistling of their wings is echoic as they take flight; there is no other species of duck that makes this sound.

So far we've done well, matching the wind with consistent, strong paddling. But I'm aware that once we go outside the headland of Tomales Beach, our next landmark, the wind may win the match. So we stop, having covered 3.5 miles, and climb up onto a ledge just above the beach, completely sheltered from the wind by trees. Here we make tea. It's quite wonderfully warm and calm where we sit, looking across the bay toward Marshall, or 10 miles down the bay, at the beautifully sculpted background, the knuckles of Bolinas Ridge behind Point Reyes Station.

Minute siskins, finches smaller than chickadees, drop down like falling cones from the tall pine trees to snap up insects off the beach. They are green with gold bars on their wings, and they have a pretty song to sing as they fly up, returning to their trees. It's protein time for siskin chicks; they'll get to eat seeds when they are strong enough and more self-sufficient. While we're sitting here, tea time has become lunch, and Martha tells us she is a volunteer in a raptor program. She has been handling a goshawk, the biggest and certainly the fiercest of all accipiters. From Martha's goshawk we move on to Shakespeare's, as I talk about the goshawk allegory that scholars have missed; a theme that runs throughout All's Well That Ends Well. In this play, Helena has the role of an austringer (one who trains goshawks). She is given a goshawk and loses it when it goes wild. She successfully reclaims her hawk by trapping it, and then she gentles it. The allusion is penetratingly apt; the goshawk is her unwilling husband.

Even as I talk, I am facing down the bay and can see a wing of white angels closing in on us from the south. They are silhouetted against the blue sky, vaguely familiar to me, and getting clearer and clearer as they close. They are rhythmically exploring a route toward us by gliding, wheeling, and soaring in perfect unison. They are a heavenly choir, silently approaching where we sit on the altar of our cathedral. Without having to beat their wings, the violent wind becomes their toy, magnifying the power of their flight—while giving us joy. We are watching 16 white pelicans.

When it's time to tackle the final 1.5 miles to Hog Island, we review the situation. First, we take a reconnaissance stroll to the headland of our beach, from where we can see Pelican Point, 1 mile ahead. Another 0.75 mile beyond that, but right out in the maelstrom in the bay, stands the round island of trees that is our goal. Second, we agree to turn back if we find the going too hard up to Pelican Point. When we reach it, we'll decide from there whether or not we'll strike out into the bay for Hog Island. With these safety factors established, we put in and tackle the waves. But very soon we find the waves are tackling us! The sea, for that's what Tomales Bay becomes in these conditions, is too powerful for us. The wind is an unforgiving Force 6 (30 mph) on the Beaufort Scale, and it's time for us to withdraw.

Going about without getting broached by a big wave is the next test, and all three kayaks make it. Now we ride the waves all the way back to Hearts Desire, and for 3.5 miles a wonderful, surging, following sea carries us and chases us home. When we land, we don't feel in the least bit chastened; we know we turned back when it would have been foolhardy not to. Both going out and coming in, we had an exhilarating day.

TRIP 7 MILLERTON PARK TO HOG ISLAND

Type	Length	Map
Strenuous day	16 miles RT to Hog Island	4, 5 & 6

Summary and Highlights

Millerton Park, with its Alan Sieroty Beach, is a delightfully sheltered spot from which to put in, or have a picnic at the tables provided, while watching the resident ospreys at their nest. At low tide it's a muddy place to put in, but knowing the tide will be up when you get back makes the trip worthwhile. On a rising tide, this is a safe spot for beginners to make the trip up to White House Pool, 3.75 miles, and come back with the falling tide (see Trip 4). For a long, full day trip, I suggest you go north, as far as Hog Island, 8 miles. For your return, catch the mid-afternoon wind and charge back from Hog Island to Millerton Point, chasing the waves and catching them all the way home.

Special Advice

Don't be put off by the wind when you come out from the wind-breaking cover of Millerton Point. Work your way into the wind and waves to get across to the Inverness Yacht Club, and then stay close to the west shore. Remember: any time a big wave approaches you from broadside, especially at an angle, which is how it usually is on this crossing, all you do is take a big bite into it with your paddle, just as it reaches you. This well-timed stroke drives you forward and serves as a momentary outrigger that braces you until the wave slides under you. Don't let the wave threaten you—use it!

How to Get There

Follow the route for Trip 4 to Olema. Continue north on Route 1 for 7 miles, passing through Point Reyes Station, and look for the sign on your left: MILLERTON POINT—ALAN SIEROTY BEACH—TOMALES BAY STATE PARK. There is not an obvious entrance to the park, but 0.25 mile before the sign, you cross over a small bridge in the middle of a tight U in the road. As you drive uphill off this bridge, there will be a right-hand bend in the road, and as you are coming out of the bend there will be a tall stand of eucalyptus trees on your left. The sign leads into this grove, where you'll find a parking area and a toilet, neither of which can be seen from the road. The park gate is open from dawn till sunset. A small wooden bridge and footpath lead from the parking lot to the picnic area and the beach. You are not allowed to camp overnight anywhere in this area of the bay.

Trip Description

Looking southwest from the beach, 0.75 mile across the bay, you can see the Inverness Store, a big, light-green, metal building. When you put in, paddle parallel to the beach. The beach is on your right for 0.25 mile, until you pass Millerton Point. There is one lonely bench placed on the point for hikers. As soon as you pass the point, you can see the Inverness Yacht Club, a big white building, north of the store on the west shore. It is your mark for crossing the bay to find sheltered water if you need it.

Looking northwest, up the bay to your right, you can see Hog Island, 7.5 miles away. Visibility is normally excellent over Tomales Bay, and the island sits like a small, round loaf, centered at the far end of a long table of water. You will, by the way, be paddling right up the middle of the San Andreas Fault. So if Hog Island wobbles and suddenly disappears you'll know what's happening; I suggest you stay in your kayak.

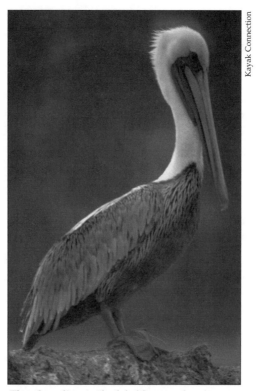

That the pelican's "beak holds more than its belly can" might contribute to its air of "comic wisdom"

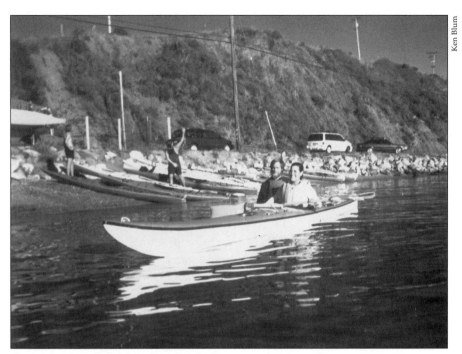

Ken Blum

Setting out from Tamal Saka into Tomales Bay

On calm days it's pleasant to have a half mile of open water either side of you as you paddle down the center of the bay. If you want to stop, there are a few decent spots on the east shore; one is Marconi (or Phalarope) Cove, exactly 3 miles north of Millerton Point, and the next is Marshall, 1.5 miles farther. The narrow beach at Marshall is easily spotted because Ken Blum runs his Tamal Saka Tomales Bay Kayaking operation there (415) 663-1743. You'll see many kayaks on their racks on the road beside this beach, and on the weekends there's lots of activity on the beach itself. After that, along the east shore, there is not much that isn't private property until you get up to Nicks Cove, 3.5 miles, opposite Hog Island.

Nicks Cove is the most heavily used access to the bay; it has two boat ramps, lots of solid concrete, and no beach. It is, however, a good place for parking, and even on a busy day you can squeeze your way in among the motorized craft to put in. Just don't expect anyone to make room for you. Nicks Cove is a useful place to leave a second vehicle if you want to travel the length of the bay in one direction only. I do this sometimes when there's a really high wind and I want to surf down to White House Pool with a friend. It's a glorious 12-mile run that can be covered in two hours.

If you intend to go from Millerton to Hog Island and back in one day, that's 16 miles. Start from Millerton Point, no matter what the tide is doing, because the wind's influence on your kayak is far greater than the tidal current's. And, throughout the trip many sand beaches are available for resting on the west shore. Indian Beach makes an ideal half-time break, going either way, and swimming off all the west-shore beaches is safe and clean.

Circling around Hog Island and Duck Island is always worthwhile, even if you don't make a landing, because you never know what you'll see. No matter which way the wind is blowing, there is always a calm, lee shore on one side of the islands for you to hang out and relax. Hog Island has a long sandbar on its east flank. Seals haul out, cormorants hang their wings out to dry, and brown pelicans enjoy their refulgent hours year round on this ledge. You'll hear the resonant singing of house finches that breed in the tall pine trees, while spotted sandpipers search the littoral for food, always bobbing their tails.

At one time Hog Island had a hog farm on it; to this day it lacks grass or undergrowth, so that I envisage the hogs devouring everything, including all roots except those of the biggest trees. It does have trees—tall, sparsely branched, wind-worn pine trees that sigh and groan all night at their long and lonely exposure to the weather. It's a spooky place to sleep out; having tried it once, many years ago, I prefer the sheltered coves on the west shore of the bay.

By day, it's a different story because you can stay only a few minutes and move on; or, if you find something special to investigate, you can linger there. I see people who spend an entire low tide exploring a tidal rock pool, paying as much attention to its inhabitants as I do when I discover a bird breeding in a place I didn't expect to find it.

—•—≡◊≡—•—

In the spring of 1997, I arrived in the shallow horseshoe cove on the southeast side of Hog Island, having come the 8 miles from Millerton, and was greeted by the raucous piping of a black oystercatcher. It flew around me, yelling at me to go away, I thought, as it circled several times. In 15 years of paddling Tomales Bay, I'd only seen this bird on the rugged rocks at the mouth of the bay. But here it was, on Hog Island, and I was thrilled. Having made its protest, it landed on the sheltered beach about 40 yards ahead of me. So I moved the kayak very slowly, without using the paddle, by pushing off the sand with my hands, until it was lodged on the sand. Then I got out my binoculars.

While I was doing this, the oystercatcher took off again and flew around me, as before, but now filling the airwaves with its entire repertoire of vocalized nuptial passion. Now, I knew it wasn't me the bird was castigating for coming here; he was a male bird persistently serenading his partner, and she must be near. I followed the bird in flight, through my glasses, and watched him land. He was impressive: a large black shorebird, with a long, thick, crimson beak so strong that it can pry open an oyster. In contrast, his sturdy legs, on which he braces himself on the roughest wave-swept rocks along this Pacific coast, were a surprisingly delicate pink.

With the passionate pilgrim standing silently in front of me, I was wondering where his partner could be when my bird made his move. He ran a short way over the sand, with wings all aflutter, and jumped right onto the back of his mate. She had been standing still and mute throughout his entire performance, so still that I hadn't seen her. There they stood, the oddest sight: two big, black birds, both facing the same way, with one atop the other. Both of them were being supported by the lower bird's sturdy, pink legs; and although they both stood at full leg-length, their thick knees stood out. Then the top bird crouched a little, and they copulated. I've seen terns do so many times, but with terns it looks more natural because their legs are so short that they are in much closer contact.

The whimsical words of Judith Wright, one of Australia's finest poets, came to mind. "Whatever the bird is, is perfect in the bird . . . Whatever the bird does is right for the bird to do."

TRIP 8 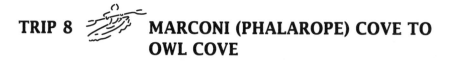 MARCONI (PHALAROPE) COVE TO OWL COVE

Type	Length	Map
Moderate full day	10 miles RT to Owl Cove	5 & 6
Easy overnight	10 miles RT to Owl Cove	5 & 6

Summary and Highlights

This small beach on the east shore, with its pebble-grit surface, is handily placed for setting out in any direction on the bay. It takes its name from the famous building on the hill behind it (out of sight from the road), which is part of the Marconi Conference Center. From here, the first radio transmissions were made across the Pacific Ocean to Hawaii, and the first transcontinental transmissions were made to Wellfleet, Massachusetts.

Putting in from this beach is convenient and clean at any state of the tide, and you can leave your vehicle overnight. The site is directly opposite Hearts Desire Beach on the west shore. A most remarkable event occurred here in the spring of 1996, when a flock of about 200 female red phalaropes settled in this cove for several days. They were exhausted and probably starving. After refueling and gaining strength, they left to continue their journey to the Arctic Circle. My friends and I now call it "Phalarope Cove."

How to Get There

Coming from the south, follow directions for Trip 7 to Millerton Park and continue 2.85 miles north on Route 1 toward Marshall. Here, on your left you will see an open, unused, fenced property of about one acre with an abandoned small trailer. There are oyster racks and buoys directly opposite it in the bay. It is adjoined on its north end to a smaller, rough open space of scrub ground. This space offers public parking and direct access to the water. It is bordered on the north side by a closed yard fence, behind which is the first of a cluster of waterfront houses. From this parking area small fishing boats, wind surfers, and kayakers put into a well-sheltered bay. (The Marconi Conference Center sign and driveway is on the right, 250 yards beyond this put-in point.)

Coming from the north, follow directions for Trip 1 as far as the COAST GUARD sign on Bodega Ave. (9 miles from Petaluma). Turn left on Tomales Rd. and follow it for 9 miles until you reach Route 1 at Tomales. Turn left onto Route 1 and drive 7 miles to Marshall. Continue south through Marshall, past

Tony's Seafood Restaurant. In 0.5 mile after Tony's, the Marconi Conference Center sign is on your left; in another 250 yards the section of Marconi Cove where you'll put in is on your right, immediately behind the last house of the settlement on your right.

Trip Description

This route from "Phalarope Cove" up to "Owl Cove," north of White Gulch on the west shore, takes you past several prominent headlands. As you leave your put-in point and move out into the bay, look 1 mile across the water to the west shore, where Indian Beach stands out as it reflects the sunlight off its sand. Another 1.5 miles beyond this beach to your right (northwest), the headland between Sacramento Landing and Laird's Landing juts out a quarter mile into the bay. Tomales Beach, 1 mile farther, is followed by pencil-thin Pelican Point, a sand spit often occupied by "outsize pelicans . . . drying their damp gold wings on sun-lit evenings."

The poet Elizabeth Bishop was right again when she said of the brown pelicans she'd watched fishing: "Pelicans crash . . . like pick axes, rarely coming up with anything to show for it, and going off with humorous elbowings." From your kayak on Tomales Bay, you'll see the patience of these birds when they're fishing, too. Each pelican puts up with the company of a satellite gull that accompanies it on every fishing flight. When the pelican strikes the water, the gull immediately lands beside it. If the big brown bird does make a catch, the gull closes in to snatch up whatever fragments may fall from the pelican's mouth. In *As You Like It*, Shakespeare got it right when he wrote, "Who feeds the raven, also caters to the sparrow."

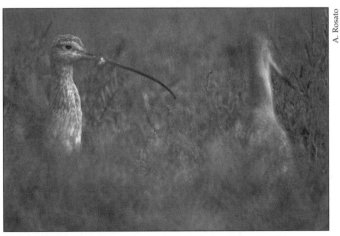

Pickleweed makes a haven for the long-billed curlew and the marbled godwit

A. Rosato

After Pelican Point, Hog Island is 0.75 mile ahead to your right (north), and to your left you begin to see into a large bay on the west shore. The bay extends a full half mile between its shoulders, and there's a sandy beach a quarter mile long at the back of it. This beach has white chalk cliffs at its north end that are unique on this shoreline. This is White Gulch, a popular environmental camping area on weekends. You are free to set up camp anywhere along this shore, and I have seen as many as three separate, large groups using the area at once. Often, in the summer months, you'll find a yacht or motor cruiser anchored in this bay, which somewhat disturbs the primordial beauty of the place. But if you paddle on another half mile along the west shore of Tomales Bay you will come to a delightful unnamed cove that I have dubbed "Owl Cove."

The first time I landed here, 15 years ago, I explored the terrain behind the cove, looking for a covert campsite, and found a wonderful place. There is a huge old pine tree with great spreading limbs sheltering the ground beneath it. Under this tree, I found a great horned owl—dead. The owl's feathers were widely scattered and its breast had been a meal for some other predator. Had the owl been jumped by a red fox or a bobcat, just as it made its own strike at a rabbit? There was rabbit fur on the ground, too.

On this trip you are practically guaranteed a good surf back to Marconi Cove, with the wind behind you from your right quarter. As you come out of Owl Cove, Nicks Cove is 1.5 miles due east, across the bay, and the wind pouring down White Gulch is coming out of the west. It is tempting to go with it, across to Nicks Cove, but if you do you'll lose its benefit for the long haul home. Once you are out of the White Gulch westerly airstream, the wind returns to its normal direction, which is more northerly.

Paddle out of Owl Cove staying on the west side of Hog Island as you head south. Look for the navigation aid—a cage on a tall steel post—between Hog Island and Pelican Point. If you paddle up to it, you can see which way and how fast the tide is moving. From here you are set for a long, downwind, diagonal run across the bay.

Two memorable days on this route demonstrate the diversity of the Tomales Bay ecology. One day involved a small, colorful, pelagic shorebird, no bigger than a starling, called a red phalarope; it winters on the oceans of the southern hemisphere, breeds in the near-Arctic tundra, and doesn't belong in the bay. The other day concerned a snake, as colorful as a harlequin, that does belong here, and would like to pass unnoticed.

In May of 1996, as the vanguard of the red phalarope population (all the female birds) was migrating far offshore, heading for the Arctic Circle, there was a hunger crisis. Timing their long flight two weeks ahead of the male birds, to stake out their nesting sites, these birds experienced a critical shortage of minute jellyfish, tiny fishes and crustaceans that should have been fueling them. Many thousands of them survived by coming to shore and finding sheltered bays, where they could add insects to their menu and recover their strength. Normally, we seldom see these birds when the females are in their wonderful full red plumage as they fly north. We only see a few stragglers in their gray plumage, on their way south. These are usually juveniles that have gone astray.

Imagine, then, the incredible experience of putting in at Marconi Cove, where my wife and I found ourselves weaving a path through at least 200 of these extraordinary little birds. They were so tame and purposeful in their feeding that they made no effort to get out of our way. Almost all of them were females: truly red over their whole body and wings, with black heads and faces, but with bright white cheeks and yellow bills. They sat high on the water, as all phalaropes do, swimming and spinning as though invisibly pivoted, while pecking at the surface of the water for minutiae, without pause. They were too busy to notice us. This is why Marconi Cove is otherwise known as Phalarope Cove.

The day of the snake was in the spring of 1997 when three of us set out for Hog Island from Phalarope Cove and stopped for lunch at Tomales Beach on the west shore. We'd finished eating and were going to move on when Justin, who is a natural fossil-finder, studying archaeology at San Francisco State University, signaled us to join him. Obviously, he'd found something special, so Sanna and I closed in. He was standing where the edge of the undergrowth met the hot sand. A narrow belt of shade spread over the last bit of sand; in this strip of shade was the most beautiful snake I have ever seen.

It looked up at us with its black eyes, and its tongue darted in and out of its mouth, testing the atmosphere altered by our presence. It was about 30 inches long and slender, no thicker than my forefinger, with a scaled head only slightly bigger than its body's circumference. But its color design was so rich and elegant that we described all the details of it to each other, just to make sure each one of us was seeing what we thought we saw. Its basic color was black, shiny, anthracite black. Extending along the full length of its back was a ribbon of red, and this band was like a continuous blurry line of the letter RRRRRRRRR as I type it here. Along both its flanks there was a lovely line of blue, sky blue, like two narrow racing stripes. And its belly was a pale creamy blue. There was nothing venomous about this snake.

━━ ⊠◊⊠ ━━

TRIP 9 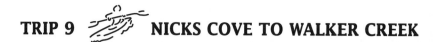 NICKS COVE TO WALKER CREEK

Type	Length	Map
Moderate half day	9 miles RT to Walker Creek	6
Easy half day	7 miles RT to Walker Creek Bridge	6

Summary and Highlights

Nicks Cove is the nickname of Miller Park, the major public fishing access to Tomales Bay. Walker Creek is the second freshwater source for the bay, after Papermill Creek. Timed carefully with the tides, this trip is the perfect afternoon-evening canoe or kayak paddle. More than one canoe, or two single kayaks, would crowd the upper reach of the creek. Company invites conversation, and disturbs the silence essential to recognizing every sound of nature: a deer coughing, a fish jumping, kingfishers rattling, an oriole calling its own name, and a warbling vireo warbling. Passing under the Route 1 bridge over Walker Creek, you enter a private, riparian world that is hard to match anywhere in California. There aren't many places like this left unspoiled. Go there quietly—alone, or with your best friend.

Special Advice

Three quarters of the route, from Nicks Cove as far as the Route 1 bridge (3.5 miles), is suitable for a small group. You need the top hours of a 6′ 2″ tide to ensure a good passage there and back. Higher tides automatically give you a wider time frame for the trip. If you are going farther than the bridge, allow yourself at least two hours either side of high tide. Do not go under the Route 1 bridge in a group. If you do, your trip will become an intrusion into a sanctuary that deserves minimum impact as much as it deserves to be seen. The land either side of the upper creek is strictly private, and jealously guarded. Please do not make a landing, and thereby upset the landholders.

How to Get There

Follow directions for Trip 1 for 9.6 miles from Petaluma to the COAST GUARD sign at the junction of Tomales Rd. with Bodega Ave. Turn on Tomales Rd. and follow it for 9 miles until you reach Shoreline Highway (Route 1). Turn left onto Route 1. In 0.85 mile you'll cross the bridge over Walker Creek. The creek will now be on your right for 1 mile; then turn away from it to start climbing onto higher ground. In 1.5 miles beyond the bridge, there will be a scenic overlook with a rounded, blacktop rim separating it from the road. Since there is no break in the rim, drive over it and park to get a fine overview of the Walker Creek delta as it spreads out into Tomales Bay. This reconnaissance will prove helpful: it shows you the layout for the navigable channel, which is hard to identify from your kayak.

1.3 miles from this turnout, the entrance to Nicks Cove is on your right, tucked out of sight as you drive steeply downhill. Tall eucalyptus trees to your right screen the entrance, and you may see vehicles parked in the wood. If you miss the entrance, you will see Nicks Oyster Bar on your right. Stop, and you will see the entrance to Nicks Cove behind you. The official designation for this cove is now visible: MILLER PARK—Public Fishing Access— Open 5 A.M. to 10 P.M. There is a $5/day-use fee for parking in the paved area or in the woods. To park overnight, at no extra charge, your vehicle must be parked in the woods above and behind the parking lot.

From the south, follow directions for Trip 8 on Route 1 as far as Marconi Cove, and continue north through Marshall. About 3.5 miles beyond the MARSHALL town sign, Nicks Oyster Bar and the MILLER PARK (Nicks Cove) sign are on your left. It is worth driving 1.3 miles north of Nicks Cove to use the scenic overlook, on your left, for a look at the Walker Creek delta.

Trip Description

There are two concrete boat ramps and no beach at Nicks Cove. Putting in can be rough when the onshore breeze sends small waves toward the launch ramps. Use the dock between the two ramps for putting in only if you are not hindering bigger craft users. Since there's a lot of seaweed around I use it to make a seal-launch pad and simply slide down it into the water. Unlike a seal I slide in backwards, rudder first, and avoid rasping the vulnerable heel of my kayak on the cruel concrete. If you seal-launch backwards, the rear half of your kayak carries all the craft's weight before it is off the seaweed pad, and the curvature of the bow doesn't allow it to grate on the concrete as you float off.

A small breakwater protects the boat ramps; as soon as you are clear of it, turn north for Preston Point, 1 mile away. Ahead there is a prominent feature, a cedar tree on the left of a stand of tall eucalyptus trees, overlooking the Walker Creek delta. And there is a pyramid-shaped knoll behind these trees. A half-mile from Nicks Cove on the shore to your right, you'll see a small group of derelict cabins, all supported over the flood marsh on stilts. One of them has fallen over and stands absurdly on its roof. The group of buildings is named Hamlet on the map. The place doesn't look much like Elsinore to me, but perhaps the prince is in the house that's upside down.

Ahead, on your left, you'll see the remains of oyster racks. Stay well to the right of them, and look out for a 3" diameter, yellow plastic post, which is on a line between Nicks Cove and Preston Point. Paddle toward this post and work your way around the mudflats on your right. If you have planned your trip properly, the water will be shallow enough for your paddles to be touching bottom with every stroke, for a while. But it is definitely navigable.

When you have come a full mile, and are about 200 yards away from Preston Point, you will see the main channel into Walker Creek on your right. It's quite broad and has plenty of water. Route 1 is on your right, running closely parallel to the creek. Soon, you'll paddle past five rusty steel columns that must have carried a substantial bridge across the creek at one time; and, ahead to your left, there's an impressively steep, 500-foot-high hill, like a closed fist with knuckles, looming above you. One of the good reasons for making this an evening trip is that then the sun is behind you, making visibility excellent. Another is that the cool evening endorses the calmness of the creek.

After 1.75 miles in the creek you pass under a narrow, old bridge that leads to Camp Tomales, on your left. The creek, which has all this time been broad enough to look like a river, now makes a loop. Stemphl Creek enters Walker Creek discreetly from your left. As you come out of the loop, unexpectedly close in front of you is the modern, concrete bridge that carries Route 1. Under the bridge are scores of mud nests, glued to the smooth concrete by cliff swallows. The water is shallow, and the creek has become a creek, rather than a river.

At this point you are 3.5 miles from Nicks Cove; and, if in a group, you should go no farther. But if you are going solo, or with one friend, press on into a sanctuary such as you will only find described in great poetry. (Try Geoffrey Chaucer's lines from *The Parliament of Fowls*: "The air of that place

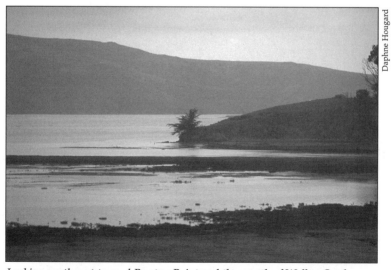

Looking northwest toward Preston Point and the mouth of Walker Creek

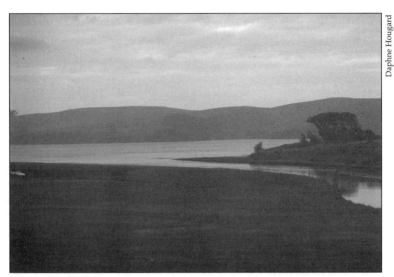

Daphne Hougard

The southwest view of Preston Point and the mouth of Walker Creek

was so temperate that there was no imbalance between hot and cold.") Watch the current because, if it's not going with you, your time frame for completing the trip is running out. If it is still going with you when you get this far, you'll not be stranded. You have another mile of fairly narrow, but easily navigable, water ahead, before the foliage from both banks of the creek closes in and bars your way.

On the last day in June, with a 6' 5" tide, flooding at 9 p.m., I had an excellent opportunity to put in at Nicks Cove and explore Walker Creek. I'd been warned that a ferocious farmer, whom I'll call the Green Knight, might decapitate anyone he found on the creek in his territory. As it was, he had already strung barbed wire across the creek as a warning of his wrath.

I'd spoken with the landlord neighbor of this belligerent, and he was cordial with his explanation of the right of way. "It's a tidal creek, open to public use so long as it's tidal." It gave him pleasure to see a kayak or canoe passing by his house. He said that legal advice on the right of way had been sought by some people, and, on the strength of the advice given, the barbed wire had been cut. Not by the farmer.

Armed with wire cutters, I tested the waters passing through the domain of the intimidating Green Knight. As I approached Preston Point, the signs were propi-

tious. An honor guard of 14 white pelicans, 12 great white egrets and about a hundred Caspian terns was standing at the delta entrance to the creek. With cautious strokes I paddled past them. And none moved.

It was after 7 p.m., and the steep hill towering over me cast deep shadows as I glided along. For a while Route 1 was so close to me that when a car came by it was as if we were using the same highway; only my lane was slightly lower than the overtaking car's. Passing under the Route 1 bridge, I saw that all the cliff swallows' nests were empty, though large numbers of immature swallows were insect hawking in the area. Perhaps they are still roosting in their nests at night, I thought, as I paddled on.

The creek was patrolled by kingfishers, many of them, with much vocal rattling. I saw the home of the man who'd been cordial to me, which was set well back from the creek on higher ground. It had a group of lofty cedar trees around it, and there were sheep grazing down to the water's edge. After passing this property, I knew I would soon encounter the barbed-wire barrier. Would it be up, or down? Sure enough, new stakes were in place to hold the wire. But on both sides of the creek, the wire had been cut and wrapped around the stakes. The way was clear, so I glided on until the growth of trees and fallen limbs blocked the way.

Talking of territory and property: the loveliest example of these concepts that I saw, all evening, was the nest of a northern oriole. It was a "finely woven basket" of lichens, hanging over the water; exactly as the Audubon Field Guide for Birds describes it.

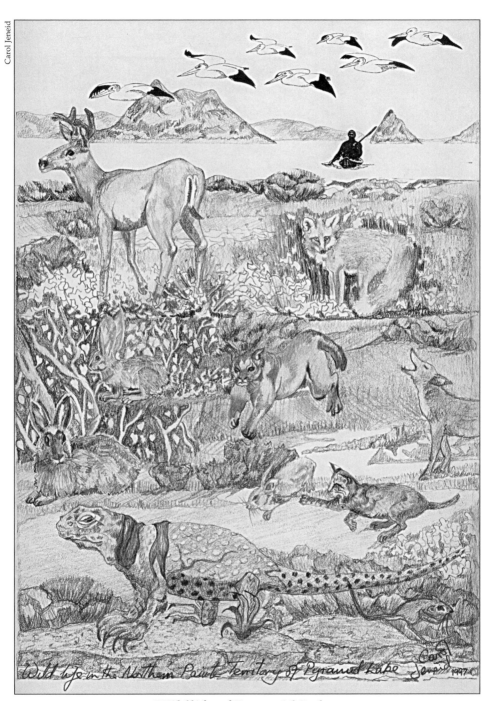

Wildlife of Pyramid Lake

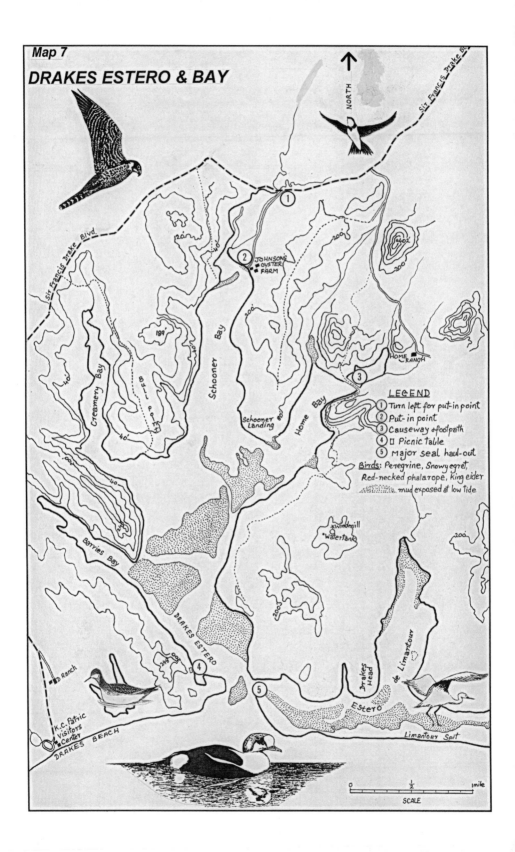

Map 7

DRAKES ESTERO & BAY

NORTH

Sir Francis Drake Blvd.

Sir Francis Drake Blvd.

1400'

200'

200'

200'

JOHNSONS
OYSTER
FARM

Creamery Bay

Bull Point

180'

200'

40'

40'

40'

40'

40'

Schooner Bay

Schooner
Landing

Home Bay

HOME
RANCH

LEGEND
1 Turn left for put-in point
2 Put-in point
3 Causeway & footpath
4 □ Picnic table
5 Major seal haul-out
Birds: Peregrine, Snowy egret,
Red-necked phalarope, King eider
.... mud exposed at low tide

Berries Bay

40'

40'

40'

×windmill
•watertank

200'

200'

200'

Drakes Head

de Limantour

Estero

DRAKES ESTERO

200' 200'

□ 4

5

■ Ranch

K.C. Patric
Visitors
Center

DRAKES BEACH

Estero

Limantour Spit

0   ½   1 mile

SCALE

Chapter 5

West of Tomales Bay

TRIP 10 DRAKES ESTERO AND ESTERO DE LIMANTOUR: From Johnson's Oyster Farm

Type	Length	Map
Easy half day	5 miles RT to Creamery Bay	7
Easy day	7 miles RT to esteros' shared seamouth	7
Moderate full day	13-15 miles RT with Limantour options	7

Summary and Highlights

Enter Drakes Estero from Johnson's Oyster Farm, 3.5 miles inland from the ocean. Mr. Johnson came back as a young man from the Korean War in 1953 and started his oyster farm. His operation uses a great deal of Schooner Bay, and over the years he has been responsible for a few million good meals eaten by people who have never been near Drakes Bay. He's also responsible for a few million blue plastic caps washed up around the shores of the estero—items necessary to his farming process that get washed or thrown away. They are the only items despoiling an otherwise wonderful body of water.

The two esteros, with their five major bays, and the sea channel feeding them, form a magical spread of water contained in a pastoral setting of gently rolling hills. Cows, coyotes, and silver foxes roam these hills. In the bays, harbor seals and oyster racks are everywhere. You should plan your route so as not to disturb either one. Both the oysters and the seals depend on the shifting nutrients that are controlled by the shifting tides. And kayakers, too, have to work closely with the tides to avoid getting stranded.

Special Advice

No recreational boating of any kind is permitted on these two esteros from March 15 through June 30. This is to protect the seals' pupping. From July 1, when you may start paddling these two esteros again, you will find that the new crop of young seals are extremely sensitive to approaching kayaks. They panic and charge into the water as soon as they become aware of you. Although their parents remain tolerant, they will join the melee, simply to be with their offspring. Even 100 yards is too close this early in their lives; give them a wide birth, avoiding a disturbance, viewed by the Fish and Game Department as "harassment" of wildlife.

Be aware of the state of the tide when you put in at Johnson's Oyster Farm. At the bottom of the tide, a wide expanse of empty oyster shells in the mud can cut and score your kayak, or your feet. Make sure that your feet are well protected, and that your put-in and haul-out times occur when there is enough water.

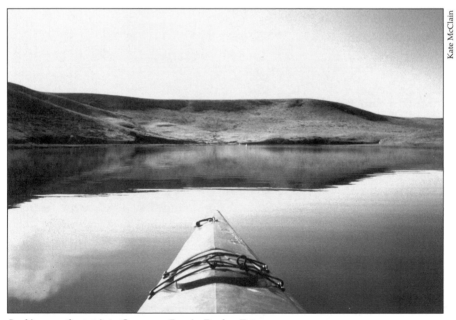

Kate McClain

Looking northwest into Creamery Bay in Drakes Estero

How to Get There

Follow the route for Trips 5 and 6 as far as the Sir Francis Drake Blvd. junction with Pierce Pt. Road. Stay on Sir Francis Drake, going west for 2.75 miles. Turn left (south) at the sign on your left, for JOHNSON'S OYSTER COMPANY—OYSTERS FOR SALE. OPEN 8.00 A.M. TO 4.30 P.M. CLOSED MONDAY. Drive 100 yards to a cattle grill, and from there continue onto a well-made road of crushed oyster shells. In 0.6 mile you reach the oyster farm. Turn right, in front of a long white fence, for free parking. There is no open or closing time for hikers or kayakers, but it is understood there is no overnight parking, and camping is not allowed anywhere on the two esteros. (The hiking in this area is excellent.)

Trip Description

On normal low tides (abnormal low tides are marked as *minus* tides in your tide book), you can reach the ocean from Johnson's Oyster Farm, but you may have to wriggle your way through mud in a few areas. With good planning, the tides present no problem at all. When the water is low, approaching oyster racks guarantees some depth, but there's a serious risk of running your kayak onto submerged metal spars.

There are left- and right-hand routes to the estero side of Drakes Beach and the two esteros' joint opening to the bay. I suggest you go south, down Schooner Bay, keeping to the west shore. After 1.5 miles you can turn right into Creamery Bay and explore that for a mile. It has lovely sloping pasture all around it, where cows used to produce an outstanding milk yield (there are fewer cows per acre these days). Or, if you pass that bay, after 2 miles you come to the opening of Barries Bay. Stick close to the point at the entrance to Barries Bay and turn northwest into the bay. That will get you around a major mud trap and into the channel for the next mile to a picnic site near the esteros' mouth.

You'll be following a line of cliffs and a rock shore on your right, and when these peter out you'll come to a shallow cove with a sandy beach. You'll see the top of a thick post set back in the sand dunes. You can see neither its base nor the nearby picnic table and fire grill. You don't see them unless you walk up the shore to explore around the post. There's always plenty of dry kindling wood lying around, and that grill is just perfect for roasting oysters on the shell. You can buy your oysters from Mr. Johnson before you put in.

From this picnic area, you've a number of options. A good one is to leave your kayaks where they are and hike south across the dunes to the ocean beach. It's one of Nature's elegant curves, miles and miles of pristine sand defining Drakes Bay. You are now standing on Drakes Beach, near the mouth of the two esteros. Go left and you'll be able to inspect the cut that separates you from Limantour Spit, through which the ocean pours in and out like a liquid hourglass. Some days the passage in this cut is very wild for a kayak and others it's very easy, depending on the wind and tide. It's well worth a reconnaissance on foot if you are thinking of putting out into the bay.

From the picnic area you can paddle 0.3 mile east and aim for the shoreline north of Limantour Spit, following that east. After 1 more mile, with Drakes Head on your left, you can then turn north and enter Limantour's largest bay. Or, instead of turning north, you can keep going east for another mile to the end of the estero. The biggest herd of harbor seals hauls out on the northern tip of Limantour Spit, so you give this point the widest berth by hugging the shore to the north of it.

The bird life you'll see along the way could include any, or all, of the West Coast loons: the Pacific loon, the red-throated loon, and the biggest loon—so improperly called the "common" loon. In England this same bird is called a great northern diver. There is a colony of white pelicans at Limantour, and these huge birds move around. They are often found at the north end of Home Bay and, at low tide, on the mud flats east of Barries Bay. Another favored spot is at the back of Home Bay. With their wingspan of 9.5 feet, the white pelican's only rival in size in North America is the California condor. Unlike the smaller brown pelicans, they never dive from the air to fish. They prefer to float in shallow water, often working together to herd the fish while ducking their heads to scoop them up.

Having approached the sea from Johnson's Oyster Farm by following the west shore, a good way to get back from the esteros' shared seamouth is by following the east shore and exploring Home Bay. When the water is low there's a lot of mud as you start to head north, and, typically, it's not visible. You can circumvent this by going 0.5 mile northwest, and then bearing northeast back to the east shore. Once you get around this big patch of mud, you can hug the east shore all the way into Home Bay. Then, cutting northwest across the bay to Schooner Landing, you go north all the way back to the oyster farm.

Make sure you do not run over oyster racks. They lie flat, just under the surface, often across your route for long stretches. You can tell where they are by the placement of the lines of poles supporting them.

➤•━ ▆◆▆ ━•➤

There are two special birds of prey in this area. One is the rough-legged hawk, which I've found breeding on the high ground around the estero, though it's more usually found breeding close to the Arctic Circle. The rough-legged is as big as the red-tailed hawk, but much less common; it hovers and quarters the ground like the white-tailed kite as it searches for small mammals. The other special raptor, an attacker rather than a searcher, is the peregrine falcon that winters here. Rough-legged hawks like unwooded territory such as they find here; as for peregrines, they like to live near large bodies of water where waterfowl and shorebirds take care of their hunger.

One windy mid-winter day, as I was returning north along the east shore, there was a male peregrine, a tiercel, standing in the air current sweeping over the bluff on my right. It made no move to avoid my approach, and so I was able to watch it for a long time before passing almost directly under it. Then it was behind me, and soon my attention focused on a female red-breasted merganser swimming ahead of me. I was plowing along into the wind, and getting a bit wet. I was making no effort to slow down to watch things, but letting them come up to me as they always will. The merganser was now only 20 yards ahead, and I was wondering why she wasn't diving to avoid me when the answer practically landed in my lap.

She pushed down with her feet to rise high in the water and then plunged under the surface, a fraction ahead of the death bolt that almost hit her. It was the peregrine that I'd been watching and had left behind me. The merganser had been watching it, too. The peregrine wanted her to fly, and she knew that. And she hadn't dived because she wouldn't know where the peregrine was when she came up. I had paddled into this standoff scenario, and when the peregrine felt frustrated he stooped at her anyway. The merganser dived because she saw death coming for her; and I got to hear the "thrumming" vibration of death's wings, and looked into its big brown eye—an eye that I know weighs about an ounce and is almost as big as my own.

TRIP 11 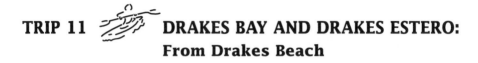 DRAKES BAY AND DRAKES ESTERO:
From Drakes Beach

Type	Length	Map
Moderate day	10 miles RT to Johnson's Oyster Farm	7
Moderate half day shuttle	5 miles one way to Johnson's Oyster Farm	7
Moderate half-to-full-day exploring	2–20 miles in Drakes Bay	7

Summary and Highlights

Drakes Bay was first called *Bahia de los Reyes*, "the Bay of The Kings," just as Point Reyes was originally called *La Punta de los Reyes*. Then along came the *Golden Hinde*, with Sir Francis Drake in charge, and he called the bay *Nova Albion*. Much later, the bay was renamed for him. Visually, the bay is a superb crescent, so well protected in the crook of its west end that it's no wonder Sir Francis secured his vessel there. The ship's sailors saw high, chalk cliffs whose undulating outline and height reminded them of the sea cliffs of Kent and Sussex.

Special Advice

In the fall, this is a perfect place for kayakers to put in for their first exposure to the open sea because the water is normally calm. But you should do so with a partner, or have a friend on the beach who watches you. Paddling offshore is very different from being on any of the bodies of water I've described so far (Trips 1–10). Look at it this way: wherever I've taken you, you could not paddle or be blown over the horizon. Now you can, and you need to remember that.

How to Get There

If you plan to do the shuttle trip, leave a car at Johnson's Oyster Farm, and put in from the beach at the Kenneth C. Patric Visitor Center at Drakes Beach. Follow directions for Trip 10 to the sign for Johnson's Oyster Farm on Sir Francis Drake Blvd. At 1 mile beyond the sign, a forest of towering steel radio masts will be on your right, and you'll begin to drive over a broad range of gently rolling hills. The landscape is on a big, open, and impressive scale. It's like driving across the Salisbury Plain to see Stonehenge, in England. This route to Drakes Bay is a lovely drive.

On your left at 1.6 miles there is a grove of old cypress trees, and beyond them you can see part of Schooner Bay in Drakes Estero. A sign, reading HISTORIC F RANCH—ESTABLISHED 1852, marks a trail that leads to a cypress grove, but there are no buildings in sight, only old cattle pens. At 2.2 miles, a sign for the Bull Point Trail and a parking lot are on your left. That trail leads to the point overlooking the entrance to Creamery Bay. At 2.75 miles there's a small sign with an arrow pointing straight ahead to Point Reyes Lighthouse. Then, at 3.3 miles, on your right you'll have a dramatic view of long lines of creaming, rolling waves—the Pacific Ocean pounding on the Point Reyes Seashore. Since you cannot see the beach the waves break on, it is very surreal.

At 4 miles, Historic E Ranch is on your left. Then, at 4.8 miles the road you are on forks, left to Drakes Beach and right to Pt. Reyes Lighthouse. Turn left. At 6 miles, Historic D Ranch is on your left, and you'll have an overview of Drakes Bay, stretching from Limantour Beach on the left toward Chimney Rock on the right. It's very windy up on the bleak, high ground. At this farm, in 1981, I saw the only scissor-tailed flycatcher that I have ever seen outside of Texas. Migrating up from Mexico, it had been thrown far off course by the wind's grip on its long, long tail. From here it's downhill for the last 0.5 mile—to the extensive parking lot by the ocean, alongside the Kenneth C. Patric Visitor Center at Drakes Beach.

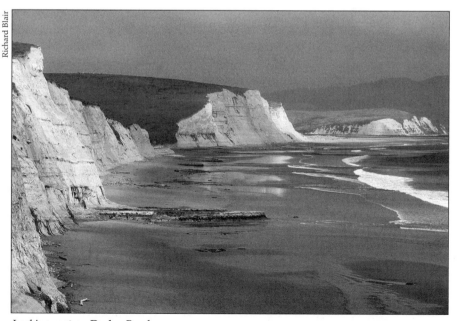

Richard Blair

Looking east on Drakes Beach

Trip Description

As long as the sea is not rough, this sand beach is perfect for putting in, and you can haul out on the sand, anywhere, for 3 miles to your right (west), or 10 miles to your left (east). Going 1.5 miles east, you can then turn due north into the two esteros, Drakes and de Limantour, and come out again. Or, if you have a second car, you can drop it off at Johnson's Oyster Farm and end your trip there.

You can't be sure what you'll do at Drakes Beach until you see the sea conditions. On many spring and summer days the sea is absolutely calm here. Small, regular waves run onto the beach and you can practice surf-zone landings with a partner. (Unless you are really competent, do not surf without a companion.) In September-October the conditions are usually perfect. But in the winter months you are going to need all the best gear: wetsuit, booties, float bag (if you can't roll), pump, and good judgment.

You'll see a huge number of waterfowl on the ocean in the winter months. Almost all of them will be hardy, diving ducks, and you would get a far better view of them from the cliffs overlooking this whole bay. If there is any chop at all in the bay, you cannot easily use your binoculars to good effect. (I don't take binoculars out to sea in my kayak.) The greatest number of species of duck I have seen in one day, at the more sheltered end of the bay, was 15. Among them were all 3 species of scoter, several harlequin drakes, and the most magnificent duck I have ever seen—a drake king eider.

The cut from the ocean into the two esteros is shallow, particularly in the center, and to avoid the pack of seals that haul out on the point of Limantour Spit, take the nearside (west) channel. The top two hours of a flooding tide are the best for a safe passage. If you attempt to enter the cut in the middle of

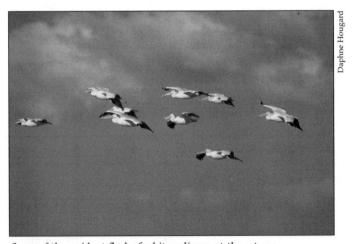

Some of the resident flock of white pelicans at the esteros

a falling tide, you'll be up against a current that's probably stronger than you are. At the bottom of a low tide, you will not get in.

The white pelicans spend more time at the east end of Estero de Limantour than anywhere else in the esteros. So if you want to explore to the east before heading north into Schooner Bay, the deeper water is on the north side of the estero. In Drakes Estero the deeper water is on the west side for 0.75 mile, then you can cut across, going northeast, to the east shore and pick up the deeper water that takes you all the way to Johnson's Oyster Farm. Or you can take the westerly route, at high or low tide, though you'll have to beware of the shallows across the entrance to Barries Bay.

❧ ≍◊≍ ❧

In early May, those tiny pelagic shorebirds the red-necked phalaropes, whose little lobed toes are just like a common coot's, are making their way up to the Arctic Circle to breed. They are seven inches long and weigh less than two ounces. They are unafraid of humans, and see us so seldom that they don't really need to be. I have seen film of a human holding the eggs of this smallest phalarope, in a cupped hand held alongside the bird's nest. When the male bird, who does all the incubating, returned to its nest, it ignored the empty nest and landed on the hand with eggs to resume incubating. Call it trust, or what you will; it is very dear.

In May 1997, I was on Drakes Beach taking a hike after kayaking there. Out on the ocean that day I'd met a number of these tiny, red-necked phalaropes spinning and pecking at the water's surface, as they do when feeding. I realized these were birds that had dropped out of the fast-flying flocks and were building their strength to carry on. Now, as I walked the beach, there was an exhausted female phalarope (I could tell her sex from her rich red neck) in front of me. She was so tired she made not the slightest effort to avoid me. Any dog coming this way would gobble her up and think about the feathers later. Seeing she had no injuries, I picked her up, hoping her to give her one last chance, out of the wind, out of the waves, and out of harm's way. She needed calm water where there would be insects on which she could feed.

There is a lovely pool, unnamed, between Drakes Estero and the parking lot at Drakes Beach. I carried the phalarope over the dunes, climbed over a fence and set her down on the water, behind a sluice gate. I could see insects everywhere, including on the water. As soon as I set her down she put her tiny feet in motion and, for the first time since I'd seen her, looked interested in life. Within a moment or two she was drinking. It was a good sign. In fact, she took several drinking pauses as she swam along. And then, to my absolute joy, she started spinning around, grabbing at tiny insects.

I know what it's like to make an arduous, elemental journey and run out of everything. I remember when I lived out of my kayak for six weeks without enough food for the effort I was making every day. Nor had I enough warm clothing, and often nothing dry to wear. This was on my route from London to Paris. When I'd almost run out of money and had no food, I still had about 20 miles to cover on the River Seine before reaching my destination in the heart of Paris, Pont Alexandre Trois.

That night I would sleep under a bridge with 20 other hobos, but if I was to sleep at all, or be strong enough to continue in the morning, I needed food. So I used my last coins to make a phone call to the Paris Bureau of a London newspaper, The Daily Express. *I spoke with a journalist, someone who'd never seen or heard of me, and I told him where I'd come from and where I was going. It worked. Nicholas Tomalin drove out to the bridge over the River Seine, where I'd told him I was bedding down. We met on the bridge, went to a cafe, ate lots of food, and drank some beer. Then I bedded down under the bridge, fortified to finish my journey—like a rescued phalarope.*

⊶ ≖✦≊ ⊷

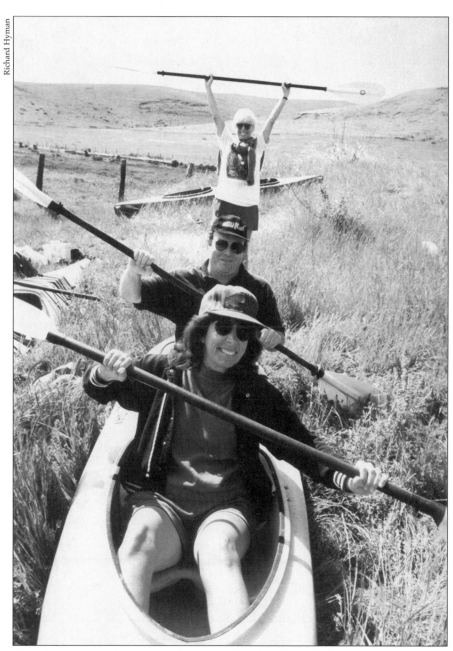

These first-time paddlers practice their form before their first launch

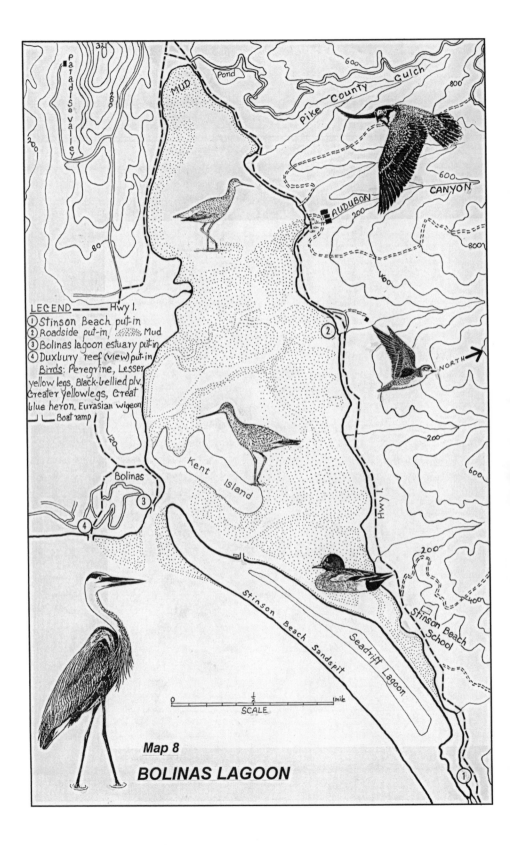

321

Paradise Valley

200

600

Pond

MUD

Pike County Gulch

800

600

CANYON

AUDUBON
200

600

800

400

80

LEGEND ──── Hwy 1.
① Stinson Beach put-in
② Roadside put-in, ∷∷∷∷ Mud
③ Bolinas lagoon estuary put-in
④ Duxbury reef (view) put-in
Birds: Peregrine, Lesser
yellow legs, Black-bellied plv.
Greater yellowlegs, Great
blue heron. Eurasian wigeon
╚══╝ Boat ramp

②

NORTH

200

600

120

Bolinas

Kent
Island

③

④

Hwy 1.

200

Stinson Beach
School

400

0   ½   1 mile
SCALE

Stinson Beach Sandspit

Seadrift Lagoon

①

Map 8

BOLINAS LAGOON

Chapter 6

South of Tomales Bay

TRIP 12 BOLINAS LAGOON

Type	Length	Map
Easy exploring	2–8 miles	8

Summary and Highlights

The late Roger Tory Peterson, for much of his long life the world's foremost bird guidebook author and illustrator, named Bolinas Lagoon in his "hot list" of the ten best places for bird watching in North America. It lies 15 miles north of the Golden Gate Bridge, as the cormorant flies. It is 1 mile wide at its broadest, and almost 4 miles long. Its narrowest section leads right up to a creek in Stinson Beach. The sea enters the lagoon from Bolinas Bay through a narrow cut between the town of Bolinas and the Stinson Beach sandspit. The sandbars at the mouth of the lagoon make this an excellent area for learning your kayak-surfing skills.

For the full length of the lagoon's inland shoreline, Route 1 runs alongside its water's edge. There are many small turnouts from which you can launch a kayak or canoe, as long as the tide is in. The lagoon is shallow, and you must work with the flooding tides. Don't forget your camera, binoculars, and bird guidebook because this is Mecca for shorebirds and waterfowl.

Special Advice

With a 5′ high tide, you have two hours either side of that peak in which to explore all of Bolinas lagoon. Better than any of the many roadside put-in

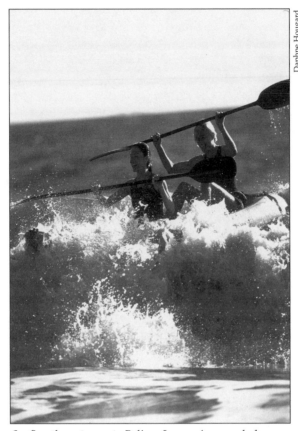

Surfing the entrance to Bolinas Lagoon in open-deck Ocean Kayaks

points is the one at the mouth of the lagoon. From here, on a rising tide the swift current will carry you straight into the safety of the lagoon. Unless you are a strong paddler, competent in swirling water, you should not try to enter the lagoon from here on a falling tide because it may take you out to sea with it. If you haul out on a falling tide, you can go with the current and run yourself up onto the beach quite easily.

How to Get There

From the south, take the STINSON BEACH exit off Route 101 and drive into Mill Valley. At the first traffic light by the Arco gas station, turn left onto Route 1. Monitor your mileage from this point. In 2 miles, at the top of a long climb, there is a fork in the road, where the Panoramic Highway branches steeply uphill to your right. It goes to Muir Woods and Stinson Beach. Ignore it. Stay on the lower road, and in 5 miles you come to Muir Beach, with the

Pelican Inn on your left. (The narrow road going left, past the inn, takes you to the Muir Beach parking lot. On Trip 13 you could end your trip there.)

Continue on Route 1 up onto a high ridge from which, looking to your right you can see large areas of violet-purple heather growing to a great size. This is an area for heather farming. To your left, along this ridge, you can see the ocean far below you. The winds on the ridge are notorious, though red-tailed hawks and ravens make it their toy. Make sure your kayaks are secure! As you come down from the ridge, Slide Ranch, a learning center for children, is on your left. In 11.3 miles you reach the Stinson Beach crossroads, with a grocery store on your right and Scott Tye's business, Off The Beach—Ocean Kayaks Ltd., in the Post Office block to your left.

For the put-in possibilities for Bolinas Lagoon, reset your odometer at the crossroads in Stinson Beach. Continue north on Route 1 toward Olema, Pt. Reyes, and Jenner. In 0.2 mile, as you are leaving Stinson, Donnie Mackin's dual business, Kayaks and Stinson Beach Health Club, is on your left.

The road between Stinson Beach and the junction with the Olema-Bolinas road, four miles ahead, is dangerous, particularly at weekends. It is narrow and has many blind corners. If you stop to put in along this road, park next to the water to avoid carrying kayaks across the road. The first good spot comes up shortly after leaving Stinson Beach, at the east end of the lagoon where open water ends and becomes a creek. At 1.8 miles there is a large parking area on the right side of the road. It has been put there for the many seal-watchers who stop to watch seals on their favorite lagoon haul out. It's an obvious put-in point, but unsuitable because of its proximity to the seals.

In 2.75 miles there's a good put-in by a section of road that has a dirt, human-made overlook. Then, in 3.4 miles, the Audubon Canyon Ranch is on your right. It is famous for the egret "rookery" and the overlook in the canyon from which you may watch the colony of nesting birds during the breeding season. At this writing, the ranch is open to visitors. Check first by calling (415) 868-9244.

In 4.3 miles, there is a crossroads sign on your right, and 100 yards beyond it a small, unmarked road crosses Route 1. By turning left here, you can make a shortcut onto the unsigned road which takes you into Bolinas, and to the estuary of the Bolinas Lagoon. (This shortage of road signs is courtesy of a Bolinas faction who don't want anyone to find the place. It is their custom to remove all signs.) In 100 yards turn left again onto the still unsigned Olema-Bolinas Road.

The lagoon will be in sight on your left for the next three-quarter mile. You cannot put in along this stretch of road without causing damage to the grasses and reeds essential for the habitat of a few Virginia rails. At 5.6 miles you reach a T-junction where the road you are on meets Horseshoe Hill Rd, coming in from the right. Turn left, and, at 5.8 miles, the Bolinas School is on your right.

To your left, looking across the marshland, there is a substantial property tucked into a small plateau in the hillside. It looks as though it's been there a long time, but it is completely modern, an exemplary example of environmentally conscious architecture. At 6 miles you climb a steep hill with a T-junction and stop sign at the top of it. Drive straight ahead down the slope and stay on the main road (Wharf Rd.) through town. Watch for the Bolinas Bakery on your right; it has good pastries and toilets you may need. At 6.75 miles, the road runs onto the beach. Here you can park and put in to go kayak surfing, birding, or fishing. First, scout the tide's rapid flow in or out of the lagoon. If you are a novice surfer, you want an incoming tide to protect you. You will quickly discover how beneficial it is.

Trip Description

Using the map, you can see how Kent Island, visible only as a sand bar when seen from your kayak or canoe, is just north of the entrance to the lagoon. If you follow the west shore and take the channel between Kent Island and the town of Bolinas, you will enter a wonderful world of marshes, pickleweed, mud bars and sand bars, with beautiful, narrow routes through them that are always navigable at the top of the tide. But you may get stuck in the mud if your timing is off. This is great territory for the canoe; in fact, for all the marsh and water north and west of Kent Island, the canoe is my craft of choice. You are out of the wind in these backwaters and, I hope, in no hurry. To paddle much farther and explore the whole lagoon, or to use the water all the way to the creek that comes in from Stinson Beach, I prefer a kayak. On windy days I want a craft that carries less wind than a canoe; that craft is a kayak.

The entire 4-mile length of the lagoon can be paddled on a 5' tide by staying close to the shore, running alongside Route 1. There's enough water over on that side to paddle in, without getting stuck, two hours before and after a 5' tide. I paddle from the creek behind my house in Stinson Beach into the lagoon and use this stretch as my daily exercise. The special thing about this lagoon is its incredibly rich bird life. In the spring and fall it is one of the best migratory feeding stopovers for shorebirds: all those sandpipers, whose dean is the long-billed curlew and whose smallest common relative is the least sandpiper, can be seen. These "wind birds," as Peter Matthiessen called them in his text for *Shorebirds of North America*, are abundant and are tolerant toward kayakers. Their low-tide, mudflat feeding frenzy dictates their behavior. They really don't have time to stop eating, and that's why we can get close to them. Besides, it's many years since this family of birds were put on the "no hunting" list; by now they have no need to be gun-shy, which also means man-shy.

Clint Graves

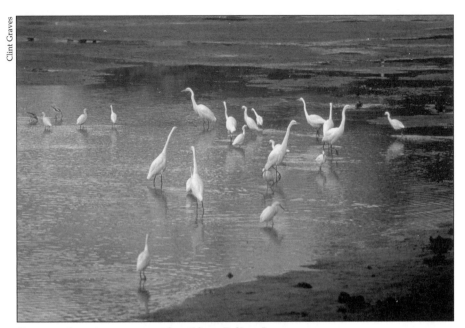

Snowy and great egrets seen at low tide on Bolinas Lagoon

The same cannot be said for the waterfowl on the lagoon. As the fall migration of shorebirds disperses, the winter waterfowl come down from the northern plains and Canada to enjoy our mild climate. The new crop of young pintails arrives first, in large numbers, followed by the rest of the surface feeders, the "dabbling" ducks: wigeon, mallard, shoveller, green-winged teal, gadwal, and always a few Eurasian wigeons. These are followed by the diving ducks, which are a bit tougher; they don't need our easy climate so soon. But all these waterfowl have this in common: they are terrified by kayaks. Our flailing paddles must look like some dreadful, low level attacking bird of prey. They can't take us, and they flee long before we're anywhere near them. The point is that they are hunted and haunted by gunfire, all their lives. They don't know that Bolinas Lagoon is that rare thing, a "safe house" for ducks. From November through February, please don't drive the waterfowl off the lagoon with your kayak, to make them land in some unprotected place.

Keith Hansen, the bird artist in Bolinas (Keith contributed his drawing of the spotted owl for Map 5), and I have seen, independently, 26 species of duck on this lagoon in the past ten years. On any winter day I can show you, from the road, 14 species. And almost every winter, in a spell of harsh weather, there are a few days with 18 species of duck present.

The tide is pouring through the channel between the town of Bolinas and the sand beach of Kent Island, flooding the backwaters of the lagoon. Hundreds of elegant terns and several species of gulls are milling in the air above the mudflats where my wife and I are quietly moving with the flow of water. We are using our paddles only to steer.

A large flock of western sandpipers, running to and fro on a blur of legs, springs from the ooze and takes flight. In tight formation, these tiny "peeping" birds sweep and swerve, rolling their bodies in perfect unison. They create a flashing scimitar of light in their flight. Curlews, whimbrels, godwits, and black-bellied plovers take off, every one of them calling its alarm. The sky is filled with the airborne riot of these larger shorebirds. But from all this frenzied flight, the dominant voices are those of the crying terns. Terns own the copyright to the sound of crisis, and they are broadcasting one now.

Carol and I, in our small river kayaks, are drifting into the heart of the lagoon's wildlife, carried on the flood into a region that cannot be observed from dry land. Overhead is this chaotic disturbance of birds, and we both know that the cause of all the chaos is most likely a hawk. First we scan the sky and then all the flying space low over the flats, but we see nothing. Soon all the birds settle again and get on with their feeding. So we glide on, sliding over the shallows, and lodge our two kayaks side by side on a shelf of mud.

From our low vantage, almost at water level, we meet a number of sandpipers face to face. I focus my binoculars on the group closest to me and see five long-billed dowitchers and one dunlin, all resting. Behind them I can see hundreds of other sandpipers of all sizes, feeding. Through the powerful binoculars, I can identify every bird and find none among them that might surprise me. (Another time, in mid-October, we saw a rare sharp-tailed sandpiper back here, and so we always search carefully.) But just as I finish my final sweep of the area, the last thing to appear in the moving circle of images is a horizontal limb of driftwood that rises about a foot above the shallow water. Standing, motionlessly, on this perch, staring intently at something gripped in its long, bright-yellow toes, is a peregrine falcon. Around the falcon, and very close to her, all the sandpipers are busily feeding, as if they have no idea the falcon is there.

The impressive size and plumage of the bird tells me it's an adult female. Her throat and chest have a creamy bloom with a few big, dark spots down to her trousered, yellow legs. Her shoulders and mantle are dark gray with a blue haze. Her head is magnificent; it is nothing less than noble. The cere of her beak is bright yellow and her upper bill is smoky blue, curving into a wicked black sickle for tear-

ing flesh. For her sickle-shaped beak and talons, the Latin word for "sickle" gives this bird her scientific title of Falco. *Her brow and head, her nape and mustache are black as a raven's wing. With her head turned in profile to me, the one eye that I can see is like a big, dark brown, glowing bulb. She has a pallid rim of skin all around her eye that augments its size. As I watch her, I know exactly why Dante wrote of this imperial bird that she has an eye like Caesar's.*

She stares down at her prey, dead and dangling on the driftwood under her right foot. I can see no blood, but black feathers just showing, etched under the bird's wing. Out of all that chaos that we'd watched, the falcon's victim was a black-bellied plover. This is the shorebird that gets its name from pluvialis, *Latin for "rain," because Pliny said it only cries when there's going to be rain.*

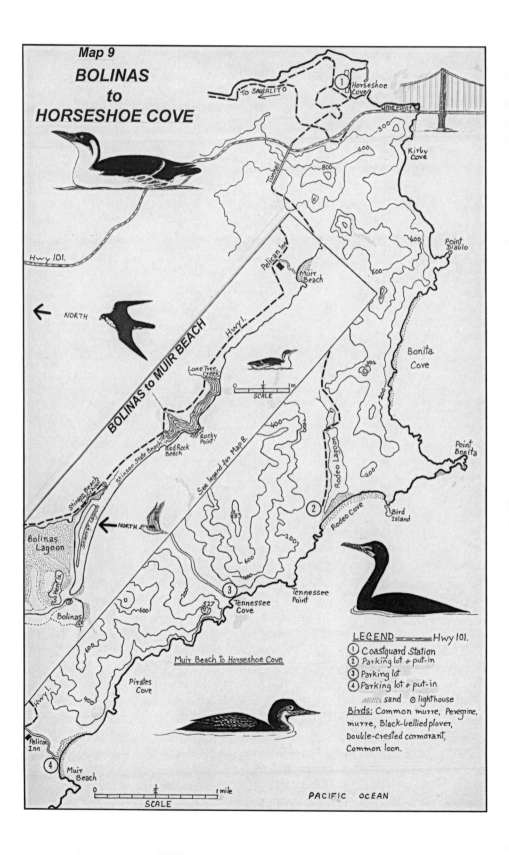

Map 9

BOLINAS
to
HORSESHOE COVE

To SAUSALITO

1 Horseshoe Cove

Lime Point

300

Kirby Cove

600

800

Tunnel

Point Diablo

400

600

Hwy 101.

Pelican Inn

Muir Beach

← NORTH

Hwy 1.

Bonita Cove

BOLINAS TO MUIR BEACH

Lone Tree Creek

394

200

0   1m
SCALE

Rocky Point

400

600

Red Rock Beach

Stinson State Beach

See legend for Map 8.

Point Bonita

Stinson Beach School

Rodeo Lagoon

200

2

Rodeo Cove

Bird Island

← NORTH

Bolinas Lagoon

883

600

200

Kent Is.

Tennessee Point

600

527

3

Tennessee Cove

Bolinas

600

600

Muir Beach to Horseshoe Cove

Pirates Cove

400

Hwy 1.

Pelican Inn

4

Muir Beach

0   ½   1 mile
SCALE

LEGEND ══════ Hwy 101.
1 Coastguard Station
2 Parking lot & put-in
3 Parking lot
4 Parking lot & put-in
░░░ sand   ⊙ lighthouse
Birds: Common murre, Peregrine,
murre, Black-bellied plover,
Double-crested cormorant,
Common loon.

PACIFIC OCEAN

Chapter 7

Under the Golden Gate

TRIP 13   BOLINAS TO HORSESHOE COVE

Type	Length	Map
Strenuous full-day shuttle	15 miles	9 (& 8 for put-in detail)

Summary and Highlights

This trip is a coastal classic that should be paddled with a companion as competent as yourself, or in a strong group. You put in at the mouth of Bolinas Lagoon, paddle out through the surf, 15 miles down the coast, and haul out just around Lime Point, under the north end of the Golden Gate Bridge, at Horseshoe Cove. When you reach Muir Beach (8 miles) or Rodeo Beach (11 miles) you can haul out if things aren't going well for you. The route is spectacular: you can see the Bay Area in the distance from the start. But it's hard to identify your position, sitting at sea level in your kayak. You are looking down the coast from a quarter to a half mile out from the land, and the only features you can clearly recognize are those promontories that jut out from the land. You move down the coast a few miles at a time, always looking for the next promontory. These features are nicely spaced all along your route.

A bird you'll get close to out at sea that you don't often meet inside the coastline is the common murre. It's a chunky seabird that gets its name from the purring sound of its voice. One of the alcids that breed on the Farallon Islands, it will dive to avoid you, rather than fly.

Special Advice

You need to be an experienced open-sea kayaker, and comfortable with the risks you take on this trip. There is good stress here, "eustress," but that easily dissolves into "distress." So, unless you are really up to it (not just up for it) don't do it. However, if you are properly prepared—fit as well as skillful, go to it! Be sure to let a reliable friend know where you are putting in, how far you expect to go, and where your alternative haul-out beaches are.

How to Get There

Follow directions for Trip 12 to the mouth of Bolinas Lagoon, and put in where Wharf Rd. ends at the beach in Bolinas. You will need a second vehicle at Horseshoe Cove, which you can park on the waterfront in front of the Coast Guard Station. To reach Horseshoe Cove (on the U.S.G.S. map it's "Bay" not "Cove," but nobody calls it that), coming from the south over the Golden Gate Bridge, take the Alexander Ave. exit after the bridge and go downhill. As the road levels out, turn sharply right at the first opportunity. This road leads to the Coast Guard entrance to the cove. From the north, take the Sausalito exit off Route 101 and drive along the coast through the town to the Coast Guard Station.

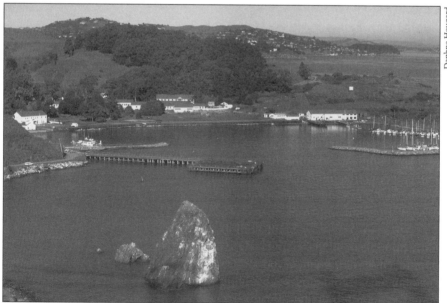

Looking down on a calm Horseshoe Cove from the Golden Gate Bridge

Trip Description

Heading southeast, along the coast from Bolinas, keep well clear of the shoreline because the prevailing swells, soon to become waves, push you inshore without your noticing. You'll have Stinson Beach on your left for over 3 miles, with Rocky Point as your first benchmark at almost 4 miles. Give it a wide birth because from Red Rock Beach, "the friendliest nudist beach in California," to Rocky Point, the sea action isn't too friendly. There's a lot of wave reflection here as the waves rebound from the rocks that have succeeded the sands of Stinson Beach. You'll be opposite the neat rows of rentable cabins above Steep Ravine Beach off Rocky Point.

Your next benchmark is the headland at the northwest end of Muir Beach. It's 3 miles beyond Rocky Point. Out of sight, around the corner, is Muir Beach, which you could find if you wanted to get off a choppy sea. I usually stop in this cove to swim, eat, and get ready for the heavy-duty half of the trip: the run down to the Golden Gate.

However, it's fun to play in the rock gardens between Rocky Point and Muir Beach. You can paddle between the many rock stacks and the cliffs along this reach, even surfing through corridors toward the cliff, with enough space to cut out from your wave before it meets the cliff. There is always an ospreys' nest to be seen here on a cliff ledge, and don't be surprised if an abalone diver suddenly surfaces near you. But there are no sea otters, only seals, in this water.

You'll see some remarkable shorebirds that feed in the impact zone where the sea pounds the rocky coast. Black oystercatchers are the prize bird among them, but the wandering tattler and the surfbird, which looks much like the black turnstone, are amazing, too. How they survive the violence of the spray, without getting knocked off the precarious perch of their pluck, I don't know.

After Muir Beach you pass Pirates Cove and then Tennessee Cove, which is a popular beach at the mouth of Tennessee Valley. Just 2.5 miles from Muir Beach you round Tennessee Point to find a half mile of sand beach in Rodeo Cove. This beach looks attractive to haul out on, but gets some big, bad waves. I was once knocked over by a good ten footer here as I came in to land for a lunch break. It was on my first run down this coast to Sausalito.

Now you have an interesting choice. If you land on Rodeo Beach, you can see at its far south end light passing between the rocky mainland and Bird Island. Do you go for the gap or around the island to reach the lighthouse on Point Bonita? If you see the gap, slipping through it makes sense and offers the excitement of exploration. But if you don't see it, you'll paddle around the island without even realizing it's there. In any case, the mileage from Tennessee Point to Point Bonita is 1.75 miles. By the time you get to Bonita you realize that you really are out in the Pacific Ocean. Rounding Point Bonita takes you well out to sea, where the slow-motion turbulence in the deep water underscores the choppy action of the surface water.

You can now head inshore and follow the long, 2-mile curve of Bonita Cove, or paddle a 1.5-mile line straight across to Point Diablo. Beyond Point Diablo you can duck into another cozy cove (Kirby), or head 1.25 miles for the inside corner of the Golden Gate Bridge and Lime Point Lighthouse, 1.25 miles head. Either way, you need to be working with the tide.

At the end of a long, offshore paddle, you don't want to argue with a Golden Gate ebbing tide. The sea comes out of San Francisco Bay with tremendous force—from 2 to 5.7 knots (that top figure is well over 6 mph). If it's with you, it sucks you along. If it's against you, full bore, you won't get through the Golden Gate. You'll have to retreat and land in little Kirby Cove, just outside the gate.

Once you pass under the Golden Gate Bridge, head left into the yacht harbor of Horseshoe Cove—it's only a half-mile away.

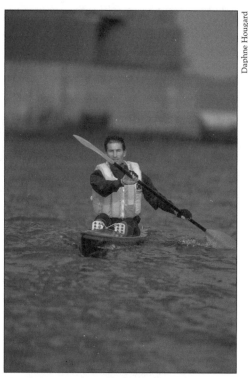

Sea Trek instructor Mitch Powers heading out to sea in his surf ski

Daphne Hougard

━━ ═◆═ ━━

The first time I did this route I was with Dennis Frolich, who was teaching the Advanced—Open Bay—Clinic at Sea Trek. He had just bought a used Arluk I and I had an Arluk II. We were going all the way from Bolinas to Schoonmaker Point in Sausalito, and had agreed to stop for lunch at Rodeo Beach. Along the way we played games among the rock stacks, surfing through narrow gaps, and generally testing each other's will. (Dennis is more than 30 years younger, and I think he was testing me.)

Since we were far offshore, we approached the beach with our backs to the running swells. I could hear Dennis yelling from way behind me to my left, but when I looked he was nowhere in sight. The yelling continued, so instead of paying attention to my approach to the beach, I looked for Dennis. I still couldn't see him, but heard him: "Look out! Look out!" And there, coming up behind me, was a wave so big I thought it was a castle wall coming at me, a wall of water that was climbing higher and higher as it closed in.

I had stopped paddling in my search for Dennis, but at least I knew he was safe behind me. I got myself going and picked up the advancing wave, or, I should say, it picked me up. For a few glorious seconds we were in sync—racing together— the wave my ride into the beach. I could see the beach ahead with people on it, but they looked like abstract figures on another planet. And then something strange was happening: we were moving so fast it was like riding a galloping horse: viscerally similar to coming down on the far side of the biggest fence on a steeplechase course.

I was literally standing in my irons, coming down, down from a great height. Only my irons weren't stirrups on a horse's saddle, but the stirrups in my kayak. I was standing on them because the kayak was almost vertical—dropping off the face of the wave—with me staying in it only by forcing my back toward the deck behind me. This is exactly how you come down from a big steeplechase jump that has an added drop-off on the landing side. You let the reins slide, straighten your legs, lean back, and more or less hope for the best.

I wasn't letting anything slide—clinging to my paddle for dear life—wondering what would come next. My paddle was ripped out of my hands and the kayak went completely vertical before plunging end over end, bow first into the sand. I had no idea which way the 18-foot kayak was facing, though still seated with my feet pressing the stirrups and my thighs bracing against the cockpit's hull. (Before I went end over end, I was automatically forcing my chest toward the deck in front of me, trying to touch the foredeck with my forehead ready for my next move.)

As I held my breath in what seemed to be the tumbler of a giant washing machine, I locked my hands flat together, spreading them wide to make as big a surface as possible. By now my actions were partly conscious, and partly reflexive because repetitions in practice become muscle memory. I swung my locked hands out to my right as far from me as possible, and immediately I got the anticipated response: upward compression from the water dynamic. It popped me up so that I could breathe and supported my whole upper body clear of the water. Holding this position, I was swept broadside toward the beach with my locked hands digging into the uplift of the wave, the one coming in behind the one that had knocked me down.

I was carried and bounced at the rush like this, all the way into the shore until I lost my hand compression in the spent wave. Then, in swirling foam, I propped myself up on one fully extended arm in the shallow water. Three little boys, who were watching the whole event, came running out into the water enthusiastically to help me. I offered them my spare arm and they pulled me upright, then hauled me in the kayak onto the beach. Meanwhile Dennis landed unscathed, and my paddle washed ashore.

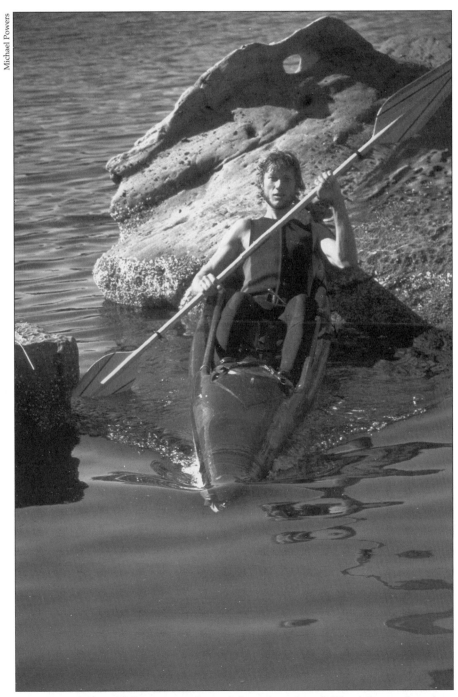

The elite surf-skier will discover amazing rock formations along California's rugged coast

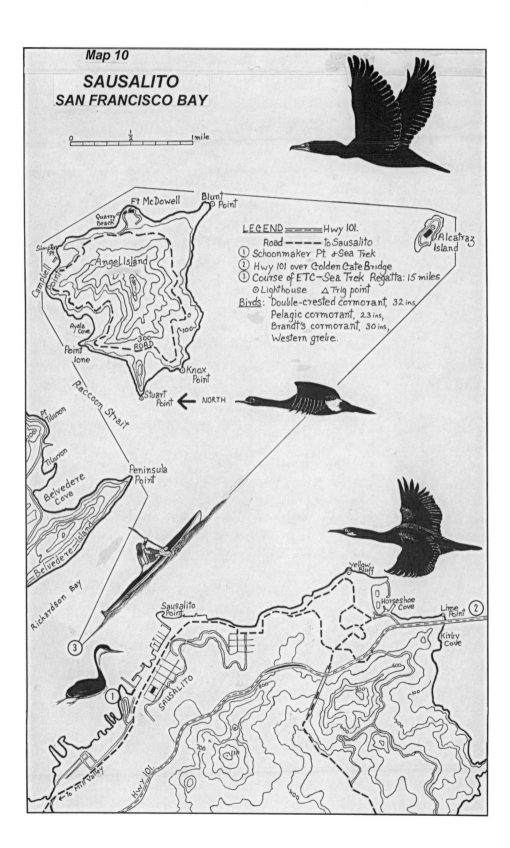

Map 10

SAUSALITO
SAN FRANCISCO BAY

0   ½   1 mile

Ft McDowell

Blunt Point

Quarry Beach

Simpton Pt.

Angel Island

Campbell Point

Alcatraz Island

LEGEND ═══ Hwy 101.
Road ─ ─ ─ to Sausalito
① Schoonmaker Pt. & Sea Trek
② Hwy 101 over Golden Gate Bridge
③ Course of ETC—Sea Trek Regatta: 15 miles
⊙ Lighthouse   △ Trig point
Birds: Double-crested cormorant, 32 ins,
Pelagic cormorant, 23 ins,
Brandt's cormorant, 30 ins,
Western grebe.

Ayala Cove

300 ROAD

Point Ione

Knox Point

Stuart Point

Raccoon Strait

← NORTH

Pt Tiburon

Tiburon

Belvedere Cove

Peninsula Point

Belvedere Island

Richardson Bay

Yellow Bluff

Horseshoe Cove

Lime Point ②

Kirby Cove

Sausalito Point

③

①

SAUSALITO

Hwy 101

To Mill Valley

Hwy 101

Chapter 8

San Francisco Bay

TRIP 14   SAUSALITO:
Alcatraz and Angel Islands Loop

Type	Length	Map
Strenuous half day (if participating in race)	15 miles RT around islands	10
Easy half day	4 miles RT to Mill Valley	10

Summary and Highlights

The beach/harbor at Schoonmaker Point, Sausalito, is in a sheltered cove easily accessible for city dwellers throughout the Bay Area. It is Sausalito's contribution to kayaking, and a prime put-in point for car-top boats. It also has the Sea Trek commercial kayaking program. Their facility and boats are just off the beach beside the harbormaster's tower. You can unload your own kayaks at the beach and then find your own parking, or make use of the Sea Trek rental and instruction program, in which case they will give you a parking permit. There is a waterfront cafe within yards of the beach.

Schoonmaker Point gives you access to all of San Francisco Bay. After putting in, you can turn left out of the harbor and head out into Richardson Bay for a 2-mile paddle up to Mill Valley below Mt. Tamalpais. Going the other way, the more experienced you are the farther you can explore; when you turn right, coming out of the harbor, all of San Francisco Bay is waiting for you, including the long course of the annual Sea Trek regatta.

Special Advice

Unless you are properly equipped and competent enough to go out on your own, I suggest you check in with Bob Licht's Sea Trek program at their Schoonmaker Beach number (415) 332-4465, before heading out into San Francisco Bay. If their message says they are closed because of bad conditions, accept it as good advice for that day. Their reservations number for rentals, tours, and all levels of instruction is (415) 488-1000. At all times in the Bay remember that big vessels are not going to get out of your way, and probably can't even see you. Also, you cannot judge how fast they are approaching over open water because, by definition, open water means there's nothing for you to use as a reference point. Follow routes that are clear of freighters, ferries, and other powerful boats. Better still, first develop your skills and get your experience with the local professionals.

How to Get There

Coming from the south over the Golden Gate Bridge, take the ALEXAN-DER AVE exit off the bridge and drive downhill through Sausalito on Bridgeway Ave. At the traffic light, 2 miles from the bridge, turn right onto Markship Way. Go steeply downhill for 40 yards, and turn right onto Liberty Way. Stay on Liberty Way for 0.25 mile to reach Schoonmaker Point Beach. You may offload kayaks at the beach, but all parking there is by permit only. Ask the Sea Trek staff for parking information.

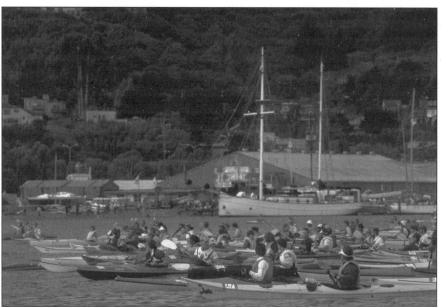

Waiting for the gun at the Sea Trek Regatta

Coming from the north on Route 101, take the MARIN CITY—SAUSALITO exit. Turn left toward Sausalito at the light. Drive under 101 and turn right onto Bridgeway at the light. Turn left at the sixth set of lights, steeply downhill onto Markship Way. Continue as if you were coming from the south.

Trip Description

A kayaking loop around Alcatraz and Angel islands, down through Raccoon Straits and back, is a measured 13.8 miles. Allow 15 miles because the tides and currents push you around. As you come out of the sanctuary of Schoonmaker Harbor into Richardson Bay, turn right and stay close enough inshore to be out of the busy channel used by large recreational vessels. Or paddle 300 yards across Richardson Bay toward Belvedere Island, and then turn right. Under calm conditions, you can then make a straight 4.5-mile run, southeast to Alcatraz. If you are not sure of the conditions, hug the Sausalito shore for 2 miles, south to Yellow Bluff Lighthouse. From there you may have a better angle to strike out for "the Rock," making good use of tide and wind. The incoming or outgoing tide will have a major effect on your progress. Coming in it will push you toward Angel Island, and going out it will drag you toward the Presidio on the south side of the Golden Gate Bridge, or under the bridge itself.

Do this trip on a day when you can catch the last two hours of the flooding tide to help you out to Alcatraz and up to Angel Island. As you come up to Alcatraz, with the island on your left, the sea's motion increases considerably as the island diverts the sea's inflowing passage and blocks its wave motion. The waves that hit the rocky shore reflect much of their energy; that "reflecto" then collides with the incoming forces, resulting in a turbulent surface. Under these conditions keep well clear of the island as you pass it because it then has a dangerous lee shore.

Having reached the east side of Alcatraz, head north. Since the island now acts as a baffle, the sea is noticeably calmer for the 2-mile run to Blunt Point Lighthouse on the southeast peninsula of Angel Island. You have 0.5 mile of sand beach on your left, followed by the 0.25-mile stretch around the Fort McDonald Quarry Point. A cove tucked in behind this point, and another 0.5 mile of sand, greet you. This is Quarry Beach, a good place to take a break, stretch your legs, and eat lunch.

After lunch, continue around the steeply wooded island, which rises to 781 feet above Quarry Beach, and make your way around Simpton Point, 0.5 mile north of Fort McDowell. Continue another 0.4 mile to Campbell Point at the northern tip of the island. Now, you can look due west and see Tiburon, 1.5 miles across Raccoon Strait, as you turn southwest toward Richardson Bay. A straight run 0.5 mile southwest will take you across the mouth of Ayala Cove to Point Ione. Now you have quite an important decision to make. The factors to be considered are the tide, the wind, the sea action, and the volume of traffic.

There are big, recreational stinkpots cruising (more often tearing) up and down Raccoon Strait. Some of these craft leave wakes that become fast-moving, powerful waves. If you take the shorter route, 1.25 miles from Point Ione to Peninsula Point on Belvedere Island, you'll be cutting diagonally across this heavy traffic lane. For half of your crossing (0.75 mile) you'll have to face off some large, unpredictable waves. Yet, if your stern's on the receiving end of the wave-makers, you can surf their signatures back to Richardson Bay.

The less threatening route back to Schoonmaker Point has you following the shoreline of Angel Island for 0.75 mile from Point Ione to Stuart Point Light-house. From there turn west for Richardson Bay, with Peninsula Point, 0.7 mile away, as your right marker. Either way, once you have Peninsula Point behind your right shoulder, you get a clear run into Richardson Bay and back to Schoonmaker Point Beach.

Nine years ago, racing in the 55-and-over age group at the annual Sea Trek Regatta, my time for the 15-mile course was 2hrs. 6mins. I was paddling my black Arluk II, in the traditional ocean kayak class. The elite kayakers, in the open class (whatever design of kayak or surf ski they choose, hoping theirs is the fastest thing on the water), cover this course in well under two hours. The course record is held by Olympic kayak racing champion Greg Barton. In 1993, after winning his two gold medals in Barcelona, Greg came to Sausalito and paddled the course in 1hr. 29mins. 18secs. This year, 1997, he broke his record, paddling a Current Designs surf ski, with 1hr. 28mins. 08secs.

What I find heart-warming about Greg Barton's participation in the Sea Trek Regatta is that this great athlete, who rates as a "best ever" in his sport, could not have been an elite track and field athlete or gymnast, though he has developed the build for that, because he has a foot disability. Well, as Kurt Hahn said when he found out he couldn't lead an athletic life: "I decided to let my disability become my opportunity." Whereupon he founded a famous school and went on to found Outward Bound and the Atlantic Colleges. So Greg Barton sat down to it and became a kayak racer. Which brings me round to the wonderful Bay Area program, Environmental Traveling Companions (ETC). They keep their sea kayaks alongside those of Sea Trek.

The Sea Trek Regatta is the premier race for kayakers on the West Coast. It is a day-long, gala event that is a major fund raiser for ETC, whose program offices are in C Block at the Fort Mason Center in San Francisco (415) 474-7662. The exec-

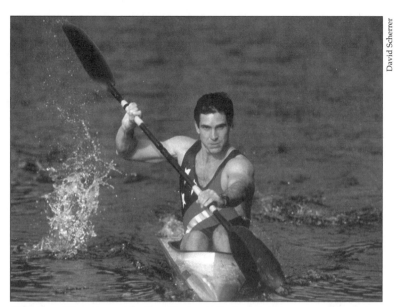

David Scherrer

With three Olympic medals, Greg Barton is the best distance racer on the water

utive director of this non-profit program is Diane Poslosky. She has two kayak projects to keep afloat: one provides adventure programs for people with financial or physical limitations; the other shares the tax-deductible proceeds from these adventures with disabled and disadvantaged people. She also has to find volunteers willing to share skills with those who cannot participate without their help.

In 1983, Diana Poslosky and Bob Licht connected through Sea Trek, and sea kayaking has become an important part of ETC's programs. The non-profit program now operates a series of summer schools on the water, including a leadership school for young people who formerly had no chance of participating, let alone helping to lead wilderness adventure trips. Anyone who has the spirit and is willing to become involved, or who would like to sponsor someone else's participation in the program, should contact the Environmental Traveling Companions' office at Fort Mason.

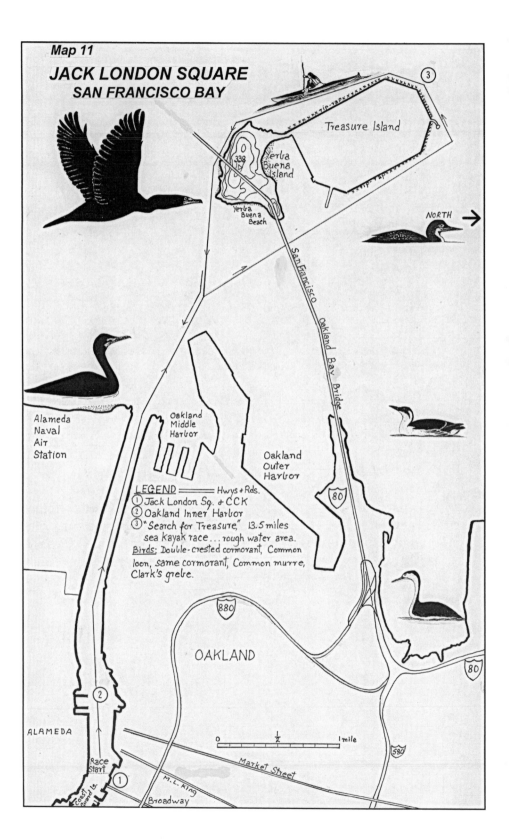

Map 11

JACK LONDON SQUARE
SAN FRANCISCO BAY

Treasure Island

Yerba Buena Island

338

Yerba Buena Beach

③

NORTH →

San Francisco Oakland Bay Bridge

Alameda Naval Air Station

Oakland Middle Harbor

Oakland Outer Harbor

80

LEGEND ════ Hwys & Rds.
① Jack London Sq. & CCK
② Oakland Inner Harbor
③ "Search for Treasure," 13.5 miles
   sea kayak race... rough water area.
Birds: Double-crested cormorant, Common
loon, same cormorant, Common murre,
Clark's grebe.

880

OAKLAND

80

②

ALAMEDA

Race Start

0   ½   1 mile

Market Street

580

M.L. King

① Coast Guard Is.

Broadway

TRIP 15 JACK LONDON SQUARE:
Bay Bridge Islands Loop

Type	Length	Map
Strenuous half day (if participating in race)	13.5 miles RT around Treasure Island	11
Moderate half day	10 miles RT to Yerba Buena Island	11
Easy half day	3.5 miles RT to Coast Guard Island	11

Summary and Highlights

The plaza of Jack London Square has a festival ambiance and is a great place to meet a friend. Good restaurants and movie theaters abound; there is a large Barnes & Noble bookstore, a great jazz club (Yoshi's), and during the summer the *Cirque du Soleil* performs here. But best of all, from the heart of Jack London Square you can embark on a variety of adventures on the waterfront of the Oakland Estuary with California Canoe and Kayak (CCK) (510) 893-7833. This is the most comprehensive sea-kayaking, river-kayaking, and canoeing center on the West Coast. Here, you can buy or rent every piece of equipment from clothing to boats, for white water, wild water, and surf-zone kayaking; touring and open-water kayak racing, and canoeing. Keith Miller and Tammy Borichevski run an instruction and rental program as well as tours from their Jack London Square kayak operation. (They have other locations in Half Moon Bay and Sacramento. See Trips 16 and 20.)

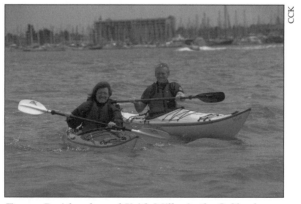

Tammy Borichevsky and Keith Miller in the Oakland Inner Harbor

If you are already set up and want to get on the water at Jack London Square, check in with CCK anyway because they will direct you to the two public put-in points and give you advice about conditions. The one at Jack London Square is from the steps (at high tide), or from the public boating dock off Broadway—100 yards north of CCKs own dock. Another, better put-in point is in Estuary Park, 0.6 mile east of CCK on Embarcadero. It is well sheltered and is ideal for less-experienced kayakers, who can head 1 mile east to Coast Guard Island. Going the other way toward Yerba Buena Island, the Bay Bridge—unglamorous as it is—has its own iron-gray authority; the entire maritime realm of San Francisco Bay is yours to survey.

Special Advice

From Jack London Square, novice paddlers should head left (east) in the Oakland Estuary toward Coast Guard Island, 3.5 miles round trip. Stronger paddlers, properly equipped with a self-rescue float, a flare signal, and a water pump, can head right (west) toward Yerba Buena Island and the Bay Bridge. Experts, only, have all of San Francisco Bay at their disposal. Pay attention to the winds and tides. Fast-moving recreational boats, ferries and cargo vessels are running set routes on their schedules; don't expect them to change direction or slow down—even if they happen to see you. Neither the natural elements nor the mechanized, commercial elements in the bay are interested in your presence.

The risk factors are entirely your own responsibility. Joining professionally led groups is the best way to go until you have enough skill and experience to make educated decisions on the water. If you want to meet and share Bay adventures with other sea kayakers, check into the Bay Area Sea Kayakers Club. BASK members have plenty of experience that they share in planning trips: call the contact person (at present Penny Wells) at (415) 457-6094.

How to Get There

Coming from the north, take Highway 580 to Highways 980-880 toward Downtown Oakland. Take the JACKSON ST. exit and turn right, onto Jackson St. Turn right on 3rd St., and left on Franklin St. California Canoe & Kayak is on the plaza in Jack London Square, at the foot of Franklin St. For the public boat dock, come down Franklin St., turn right on Embarcadero, go one block, and turn left on Broadway. The wide cement steps at the foot of Broadway are fine for putting in. If the tide has exposed the rip-rap at the bottom of the steps, there is a small dock on your right from which to put in.

Coming from the south: Take Highway 880 to the BROADWAY exit. Turn left on Broadway, left on Embarcadero, and right onto Franklin at the Plaza.

Metered parking is available on streets and in lots and garages close to the Plaza. You may unload at the public dock, and find parking. There is valet

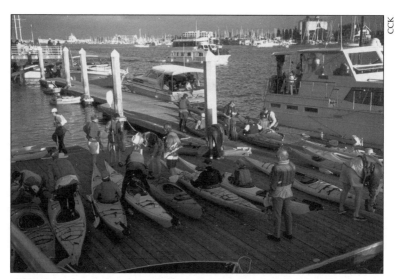

CCKs fleet of ocean kayaks ready for launching from Jack London Square

parking on the plaza in front of CCK that is discounted with a store's valida-
tion. There are restaurants, telephones, and toilet facilities all around the area.

For the less-congested, calm-water put-in point at Estuary Park (free parking 6 A.M. to 10 P.M.) head east of Jack London Square on Embarcadero. Go 0.6
mile to the park entrance on your right. The entrance is not obvious: look for
a small cement archway set to one side of the entrance. Park on the left side
of the large parking lot, near a wooden dock.

Trip Description

This is an expert's 13.5-mile route that takes you out of the Oakland
Estuary into the shipping lanes of San Francisco Bay. It's best done in a racing situation when there are many kayaks on the water (so you can be seen),
with safety vessels monitoring the route. CCK has such a race in its program
in July each year. They also offer a shorter, 10-mile course out to Yerba Buena
Beach and back, and a calm-water, 3.5-mile race around Coast Guard Island
and back. The 10 miler and the 13.5 miler are the same until the longer route
breaks to the right to circumnavigate Treasure Island. Both routes offer a fine
paddle, and the shorter one, up to Yerba Buena Beach and back, is at least of
intermediate level. It requires having self-rescue skills, carrying an emergency flare, and having someone know you are out there.

Leaving Jack London Square, you paddle northwest for almost 3 miles,
keeping the wharves not too far off your right side. Once you are clear of all
the machinery and buildings that clutter the Oakland side of the estuary's
mouth, point almost west for Yerba Buena Beach, or northwest if you are
going around Treasure Island. When you get out of the estuary into open

water there is going to be much more wind affecting you. Typically, the earlier you start, the milder the wind.

To protect yourself while circumnavigating Treasure Island, go right up to the Yerba Buena Beach and then go counterclockwise. You'd get no protection at all going clockwise until you were around the northeast corner of Treasure Island, but you would be well protected coming down the east shore.

Either way, you pass under the Bay Bridge twice, providing two visually dramatic moments. But the real drama is likely to be on the sea itself. I say "sea" deliberately because some people imagine that the word "bay" connotes safety. It does not! The water in big bays gets pushed and pulled through corridors, and converges from several directions. And that's the case on this trip: there are two areas of technically difficult water to negotiate. For this reason you should not make the extra 3.5-mile loop around Treasure Island unless you are thoroughly confident of your stamina and competence in rough water.

Both visually and viscerally, you are better off taking the right-hand, counterclockwise route, heading northeast passing under the Bay Bridge as soon as you're clear of the Oakland docks. It's a pleasant exposure to open water and a good forerunner for what's to come. You are reasonably sheltered at this point from the prevailing northwest wind that's sweeping in from the San Francisco side of the Bay Bridge. But even here the water is active enough to get your attention. Passing under the bridge you head first north and then northwest along the island's eastern shore. There is a well-protected bay on your left, curving into the island (where human-made Treasure Island and natural Yerba Buena Island meet).

You have a mile of calm water paddling northwest and parallel to Treasure Island. The northeast corner, for which you are aiming, is clearly defined because the island has been shaped into straight lines and reinforced with riprap. There's nothing pretty about it. And now, before you reach that northeast corner, is the last chance you'll have to take a drink or a break until you have rounded the whole of the north and west shores, looping back to the Bay Bridge. The day you make this trip everything could turn out to be calm and cozy, but don't expect it to be. Typically, it is nothing of the sort; expect rough water, and get out there into it. Or, if you don't want to deal with it, return the way you came.

As you turn the corner to head west, Angel Island will be dead ahead 3.2 miles to the north. Then, as you go west, you may or may not see Alcatraz Island 2.5 miles away. If the water you're in is demanding all your concentration, you won't see it. But you will see the Golden Gate Bridge, 5.5 miles away to the west. For a while now the wind and the water are likely to be very rough.

Keep a constant eye on your position relative to the riprap shoreline. Keep your distance because the wind and the wave action will both be trying to drive you onto it. Pay attention to the shape, size, and direction of the waves constantly coming at you and slapping your kayak around. Turn your bow enough to meet the bigger waves to avoid broaching, and quickly get back on course. Don't stray off course in order to have an easier time. After a good half-mile of this, things ease up for a while as you move into a lull, while heading southwest around the northwest corner of the island.

Soon, you'll be in the most interesting section of the trip. You're going to have to paddle with determination and react quickly going through a really rough potato patch. You must be self-sufficient. If you don't have a good roll you shouldn't be out here. If you do go over, and can't roll up under these conditions, leave your boat upside-down, stay with it, and ignite your flare.

This potato field (it's far more than a patch) is so demanding that you may not even notice the Bay Bridge ahead or above you. Constantly monitoring your position relative to the rip-rap shore, on your left, you may be glad to see a beach that you could aim for. There are three small beaches along the Yerba Buena shoreline as you paddle southeast alongside this island; any one of them would be worth aiming for if you were out of your boat.

With the Bay Bridge behind you, it's going to seem like a free ride home. The wind's behind you, vessels are setting up wakes that you can surf; and the Oakland wharves don't look so ugly because at least they aren't trying to turn you upside down. The huge American flag over Jack London Square is just visible 5 miles downwind. Aim for it, and it will bring you home.

The "Race for Treasure," California Canoe and Kayak's classic event, held at Jack London Square each year in July, kicks off the Bay Area's ocean-racing season for kayakers. I entered the long 13.5-mile race around Treasure Island in 1997, and pulled off third place in the traditional sea-kayak class. Bruce Von Borstal, who won this class in his Arluk I, was home in an impressive 1hr. 59mins. 19secs. These Necky boats are the best in rough sea, and it was very choppy on the north side of Treasure Island.

The short course of 10 miles—out and back to Yerba Buena Beach—attracted some of California's best paddlers, and several US National Team members. While few women participated in the 1997 race, Susan Starbird and Liz Pickens, in their Necky Nootka, placed first in the traditional sea-kayak doubles class, against all comers, with a time of 1hr. 31mins. 19secs. In a great performance, they beat out Paul McHugh of the San Francisco Chronicle—Outdoors *section, and his partner Duncan Smith, a former Navy Seal, who operates an Adventure Racing School. The men were paddling a double kayak identical to Susan and Liz's boat.*

No double boats started in the "expert" 13.5-mile course around Treasure Island. The open-class singles event was won by Brent Reitz, who came from the East Coast for the event. As a former member of the US Team, Brent's best international competition race was a sixteenth-place finish in the 1989 Wild Water World Championships.

At 40 years, Brent is still as sharp as the kayak he was paddling. He and Mike McNulty of Monterey Bay Kayaks both raced the rough Treasure Island route in their Necky Phantoms. These kayaks are 19' 6" long, weigh 26 lbs, and have a 16" beam. They are shaped like Chinese chop sticks, which doesn't explain how these two elite paddlers ripped them through the heavy chop behind Treasure Island. Their times for 13.5 miles were under two hours, with Brent setting a course record in 1hr. 53mins. 28secs.

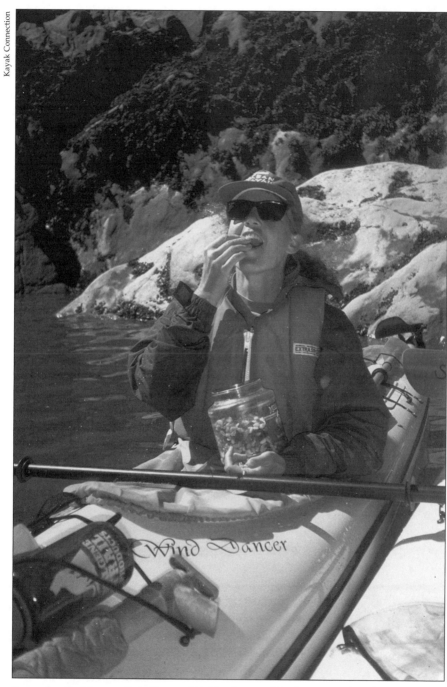

Remember, food is your fuel. Margaret Collins is one of the few to complete the 22-mile open-sea crossing of Monterey Bay

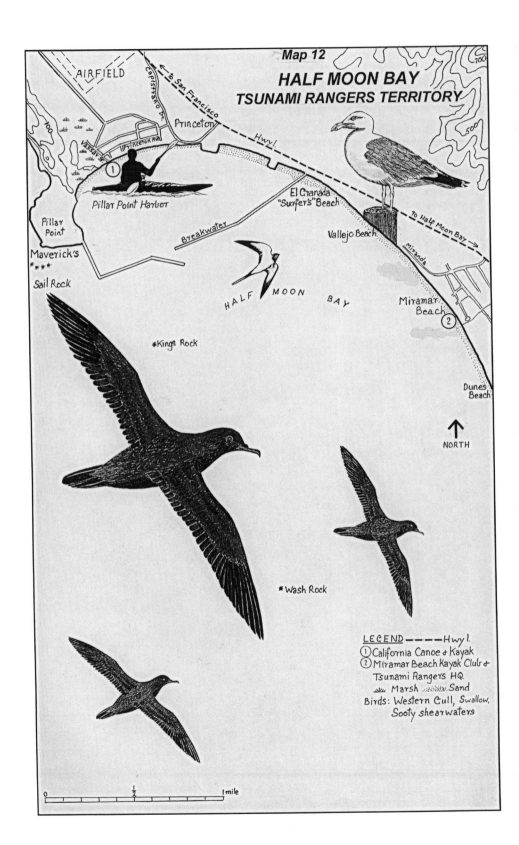

Map 12

HALF MOON BAY
TSUNAMI RANGERS TERRITORY

AIRFIELD

to San Francisco

Capistrano Dr.

Princeton

Princeton Ave.

Hwy 1.

① Pillar Point Harbor

Pillar Point

Breakwater

El Granada "Surfer's" Beach

Vallejo Beach

to Half Moon Bay

Miranda

Maverick's
* * *

Sail Rock

HALF MOON BAY

Miramar Beach
②

*Kings Rock

Dunes Beach

NORTH

*Wash Rock

LEGEND ———— Hwy l.
① California Canoe & Kayak
② Miramar Beach Kayak Club &
   Tsunami Rangers HQ.
   Marsh   Sand
Birds: Western Gull, Swallow,
       Sooty shearwaters

0   ½   1 mile

Chapter 9

Down the Coast

TRIP 16   HALF MOON BAY: A Tsunami Rangers Workshop

Type	Length	Map
Advanced (extreme)	2-day workshop	12

Summary and Highlights

Half Moon Bay is on Route 1, between San Francisco and Santa Cruz, and there are several good kayaking reasons for checking in here. The neighboring town of Princeton, with as safe a body of salt water as you can find, in its Pillar Point Harbor, is one reason. You can make use of the California Canoe & Kayak (CCK) program there for rentals and instruction (650) 728-1803, or go it alone, putting in from the same beach in the harbor that they use. The public beach of El Granada on Half Moon Bay, 0.25 mile south on Route 1, has roadside parking, and you can easily put in there. Then there is an elite team of ocean kayakers who operate out of Half Moon Bay, and who have a special range of training programs for people who want to become competent or expert offshore adventure kayakers. If you seek advanced ocean kayaking skills, the Tsunami Rangers are your role-model team of sea warriors. Trip 16 offers a unique sea-kayaking adventure training opportunity: two days, spent under instruction with some very articulate, philosophical kayakers.

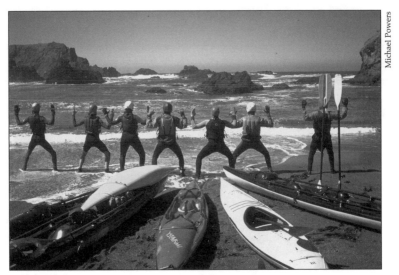

Tsunami Rangers honoring the sea with a ritual before launching at Half Moon Bay

Special Advice

This trip is suitable only for competent kayakers with good stamina. The Tsunami Rangers are extreme kayakers interested in exploring the outer and inner limits of their relationship with the ocean (their space). They use a variety of kayaks (spaceships), among them the Tsunami X-15 Scramjet, built by Jim Kakuk. For more information, contact Commander Eric Soares, P.O.Box 339, Moss Beach, CA 94038 (650) 728-5118.

How to Get There

From the north: to put in on your own or with CCK at Pillar Point (Princeton) Harbor, follow Route 1 for 30 miles south from San Francisco. With the Moss Landing Airport on your right, look for the largest shed on the airfield, marked WEST COAST AVIATION. One mile beyond this shed, turn right at the traffic light onto Capistrano Dr. Follow Capistrano 0.4 mile and turn right onto Prospect Dr. In 100 yards turn left onto Broadway and, immediately, left onto Princeton Ave. Follow Princeton 0.2 mile to Half Moon Bay Yacht Club, on your left. Turn left at the yacht club onto Vassar St. and park. On Vassar, CCK is on your left, and you are only a few yards from the sandy beach for putting in.

From the south: on Route 1, drive 6 miles north from Half Moon Bay city limit sign, and turn left at the traffic light onto Capistrano Dr. When you turn onto Capistrano, Pillar Point (Princeton) Harbor is in full view ahead of you, to your left. Follow Capistrano 0.4 mile and continue as from the north.

Alternative route from the Bay Area: Take Interstate 280 as far as the Half Moon Bay exit onto Route 92. Follow Route 92 west for 10 miles and turn right onto Route 1. Drive 4.2 miles north to the traffic light and turn left onto Capistrano Dr. Follow Capistrano for 0.4 mile and continue as from the north.

Trip Description

This trip is a course for experienced kayakers; it is a two-day intensive kayaking workshop. Depending on conditions, the course includes building surf-zone skills, paddling in heavy seas, negotiating rock gardens, and exploring sea caves. To take the course, experienced paddlers must be able to paddle 5 miles in under two hours, roll, rescue, navigate, paddle competently in 20+ mph winds, and swim 300 meters with all their sea-going gear on. Before going on the water, you'll absorb readings and videos on skills, including hand signals, kayak surfing, teamwork, and safety.

A typical first day goes like this: after inventorying equipment, the class puts in from the yacht club in Princeton Harbor and practices slalom maneuvers around the pier. This is followed by practicing signals and teamwork, and a demonstration of rolling and self-rescues. After this you paddle out into the harbor, and proceed alongside the rip-rap jetty to experience the push and pull of water and rocks. You'll feel yourself being sucked in—toward the wall of rocks—and rejected before impact. Then, on the south end of Pillar Point and just north of Ross Cove, you'll do some surfing, followed by lunch on the beach at Ross's. There you'll be debriefed on the activities so far, and plan the afternoon's itinerary. Paddling north, through the reef, to Flat Rock you'll play in the convergence of waters, and practice seal landings and launches. On the way back to Princeton Harbor, you'll group into a tight formation for debriefing.

On the second day, the course meets at Fitzgerald Marine Reserve. You'll warm up, practice rock maneuvers at the protected geosyncline, and then paddle north through the rock gardens, called by your leaders, "Sniveler's Row." Here, you'll learn how to scout, paddle, and rescue in churns, caldrons, and sea caves. After debriefing, at lunchbreak, you'll wander the corridors at Sniveler's Boneyard, where you'll lead, and receive individual instruction from Tsunami Ranger officers. At the end of the day, there is a final debriefing. One week later, all participants complete a questionnaire listing what they learned.

Eight years ago I spent a day at Moss Beach with Tsunami Rangers Jim Kakuk, Eric Soares, and Michael Powers, watching Michael's induction into the Tsunami Rangers team. Captain Kakuk and Commander Soares, the founders and senior officers of the team, were going to test Michael's all-around abilities—in and out of his kayak—in heavy seas, and in what they call "the excitement zone,"—the impact zone where waves break up on rock ledges, or beaches. The striking thing was their almost contemptuous disregard for danger combined with a very high level of performance. Giant waves came at them from all directions, propelling them in one direction, then another. Sometimes their kayaks were thrown clean out of the water by waves, always to be brought under control when they came down.

Michael, a 47-year-old photojournalist who specializes in adventure stories, spent several hours calling on all his ocean intelligence, kayaking skill, strength, courage, and endurance to find out if he was to be admitted onto the team as one of its officers, and what rank he would be awarded. The club already had a following, but only its two founders and three other men, all lieutenants, had designated rank. When the test was over we withdrew to a small restaurant for a meal and Michael's debriefing. I liked what he had to say about why he enjoys the ocean and its challenges. "Earth may be crisscrossed by man's roads and pockmarked by his industry, but the sea remains unconquered." His performance in the rescue situa-

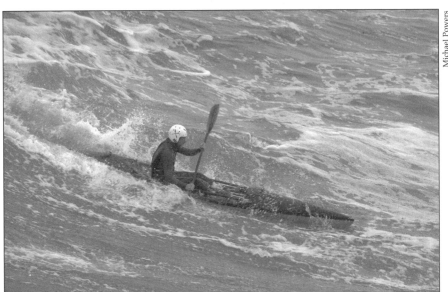

Michael Powers

Commander Eric Soares surfs a big swell in Monterey Bay

tions at the end of his arduous tests was outstanding, and he was invited to join the team with the rank of lieutenant-commander.

These kayaking commandos' techniques for mastering ocean skills are elemental. They don't think of conquering the sea because they know they can't do it, and wouldn't want to. They read the water and work with (not against) it. Often, the solution to a hazardous situation is to go under (rather than stay on top of) the water. In this way they are very like the surf scoters, black, surf-zone diving ducks that are so at home on the roughest shoreline.

If you are not ready to paddle with the Tsunami Rangers, but would like a vicarious experience with them, they've made a series of instructional and entertainment videos. One of their films, **Adventures of the** Tsunami Rangers, won Best of Show at the 1990 National Paddling Film Festival. Contact Eric Soares at (650) 728-5118 for more information.

There are great opportunities at Half Moon Bay to paddle independently or take lessons, starting with the basics and continuing into the realm of advanced kayaking. At CCK in Princeton Harbor, John Lull teaches kayaking with authority. He, too, is a Tsunami Ranger, and his 20-minute video on surf-zone kayaking is well executed, well filmed, and well explained. It is better than the commercial films I've seen. For more information about this teaching video, you can contact John by mail at: P.O. Box 564, El Granada, CA 94018.

⊷ ⇌◊⇋ ⊶

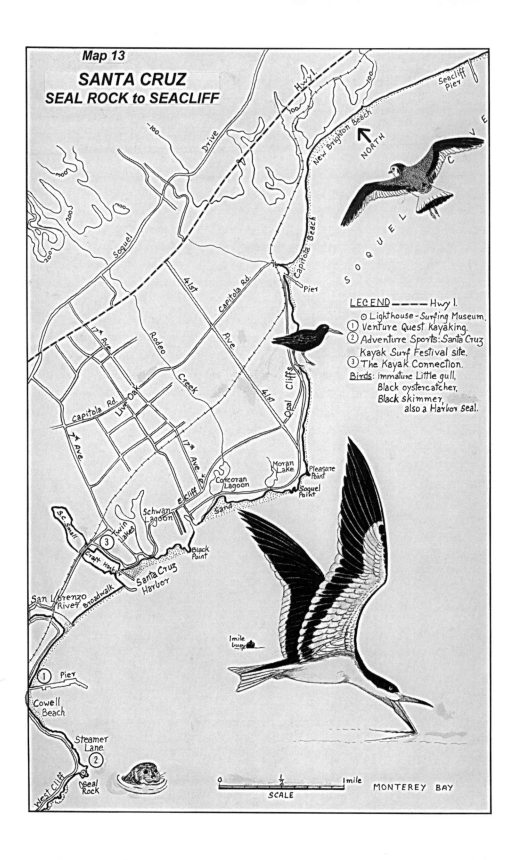

Map 13

SANTA CRUZ
SEAL ROCK to SEACLIFF

NORTH

SOQUEL AVE

LEGEND ----- Hwy 1.
◎ Lighthouse - Surfing Museum.
① Venture Quest Kayaking.
② Adventure Sports: Santa Cruz
   Kayak Surf Festival site.
③ The Kayak Connection.
Birds: immature Little gull,
   Black oystercatcher,
   Black skimmer,
   also a Harbor Seal.

Seacliff Pier

New Brighton Beach

Capitola Beach

Pier

Opal Cliffs

Moran Lake

Pleasure Point

Soquel Point

Corcoran Lagoon

Sand

Schwan Lagoon

E.Cliff Dr.

Twin Lakes

S.C. Small Craft Hbr.

Black Point

Santa Cruz Harbor

Broadwalk

San Lorenzo River

Capitola Rd.

Live Oak Ave.

17th Ave.

41st Ave.

Capitola Rd.

41st Ave.

Rodeo Creek

Soquel Drive

① Pier

Cowell Beach

Steamer Lane ②

West Cliff

Seal Rock

1 mile buoy

0   ½   1 mile
SCALE

MONTEREY BAY

TRIP 17   SANTA CRUZ:
The Sea Otter Route

Type	Length	Map
Moderate full day	10 miles RT to Seacliff Beach	13
Moderate half day	7 miles RT to Capitola Wharf	13
Easy half day	3 miles RT to Pleasure Point	13

Summary and Highlights

Santa Cruz offers a wide variety of kayaking opportunities. There are several companies in town offering rentals, instruction, and tours, but it is a great place for independent kayaking, too. The focal point for independent or commercial launching is at the harbor, in front of the Santa Cruz Harbor Office. The parking fee for "rooftop launching" is $5/car. The company with which I have worked as both naturalist and Eskimo-roll instructor is the Kayak Connection owned by Margaret Collins and Mark Pastick (408) 479-1121, on Lake Ave., above the Santa Cruz Small Craft Harbor.

Among the many trips the Kayak Connection offers from Santa Cruz Harbor is one that you can also do on your own as long as you are competent to leave the harbor and paddle close inshore, keeping clear of the impact zone. I call it "the sea otter route" because it offers a wonderful opportunity to make a kayak connection with these engaging marine mammals. They prefer to live no more than a mile from shore and spend a lot of time in the kelp beds, so you'll have no trouble finding them.

Another company in town (whose owner, Dave Johnston, can help you) is Venture Quest Kayaking at 125 Beach St., opposite the beach volleyball courts near to Santa Cruz Wharf. He also has a rental outlet on the north side of the wharf. Dave offers nature tours, rentals, and classes (408) 427-2267.

The home of the nation's leading surf-kayaking contest, the Santa Cruz Kayak Surf Festival, is also in town. The festival organizers, Virginia Wedderburn and Dennis Judson, have an on-site rolling pool at their Adventure Sports store at 303 Potrero St., No.15 (408) 458-3648. They have a comprehensive, skills-development program for kayakers. There is probably no town on the West Coast more used by kayakers and surfboarders than Santa Cruz.

Special Advice

Don't go offshore in an enclosed kayak unless you are capable of reentering your boat after a capsize. Let a friend know where you are kayaking and when you expect to return. A sit-on kayak (one that you know you can scramble back onto if you fall off) is much safer; it is easy to launch from and land on any beach. If you are using a camera or binoculars, as many people do when they go otter watching, be careful not to drop them overboard. Keep them attached to you. If they do get wet, take them to a repair shop within hours, not days.

How to Get There

The fastest route from the Bay Area to Santa Cruz is to drive south on Interstate 280. Take the SANTA CRUZ exit onto Route 17, and drive 25 miles "over the hill" to Santa Cruz. Turn south onto Route 1 at the WATSONVILLE exit. To reach the Kayak Connection and the Santa Cruz Small Craft Harbor, take the SOQUEL exit off Route 1, and turn left at the traffic light. Go 0.1 mile before turning right at the next light, onto 17th Ave. Turn right at the light onto East Cliff Dr. Follow East Cliff around Schwan Lagoon and turn right onto 7th Ave. Go up the hill and turn left at the next light onto Eaton St. Go a short distance downhill and, just before the harbor bridge, turn left onto Lake Avenue. The Kayak Connection is 200 yards along Lake Avenue on your right. 100 yards beyond it, to the right, is the ramp leading down to the harbor parking and the public boat ramp. Pay a $5 launching fee at the harbor office building (like a small lighthouse, gray with white trim) overlooking the harbor.

The scenic route from San Francisco to Santa Cruz is to drive south on Route 1 to the SOQUEL exit and turn onto 17th Ave., as before. Coming to Santa Cruz from the south, use Route 1 and exit at 41st St. CAPITOLA. Turn left at the light onto 41st St. and drive to the end of it. Turn right on Portola Rd. Portola becomes East Cliff Dr. after you reach the junction with 17th Ave. Stay on East Cliff Dr. and follow the route already described.

Trip Description

If you want to warm up before leaving the Santa Cruz Small Craft Harbor, you can turn right from the boat ramp, go under the harbor bridge, and paddle a full, half mile inland. In completely calm water, you can check out the entire residential fleet, meet a few loons and western grebes "up close and personal," and even see a great blue heron's nest, high over the harbor, in the eucalyptus trees on the south bank. I often do this warm up before going out to sea. This mini-route is just right for any first-time-out kayaker, not ready to leave the harbor.

As you leave the boat ramp, Aldo's Restaurant is directly opposite, across the harbor. A crab omelet here makes a great kayaker's breakfast, and you

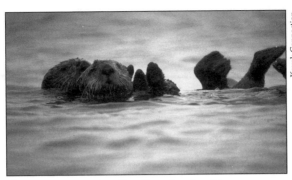

Sea otters are a major attraction when kayaking near Santa Cruz

should consider it because the sea otters you'll be seeing eat crab for breakfast, lunch, and dinner. Turning left toward the harbor mouth, you must be aware of the channel buoys and the right of way of all the motor vessels in the channel. The harbor has a long rip-rap sea wall on both sides, but the starboard (right) side wall is considerably longer than the one on the port side. If you stick to the right side, you'll encounter more turbulence in the water leaving the harbor than you would to your left. At the same time, it's more fun. However, vessels coming into the harbor from that side—some of them approaching very fast—cannot see you until the last moment of their approach. Be careful!

There's a one-mile buoy off the harbor mouth, and if you are an experienced kayaker you may want to paddle out to it, if only to look at the sea lions lounging on it, and falling off it, as it sways and lurches like some great, oval, omni-directional rocking chair. Don't go too close when you round it because the ocean swells can carry you right onto it, without ceremony. There is a territorial mood among the sea lions that climb aboard this buoy, and they don't like you in their space. I'd say 100 yards is close enough.

Whether you go out to the buoy or not, it's best to paddle far enough offshore to avoid swells that might carry you into the surf, before you head down the coast 1.5 miles east toward Soquel and Pleasure points. You're going to find two remarkable territorial species in the water off Pleasure Point; in each, the males are usually bigger than the females. The smaller of the two species is out in the huge beds of kelp, benign, curious and endearing, busily cracking shells of whatever tasty crustaceans they have brought to the surface; the others are cracking the waves toward the beach, and are aggressive, incurious, and not fond of kayakers. So, though you are welcome to approach the sea otters, with caution, stay away from the others. You know whom.

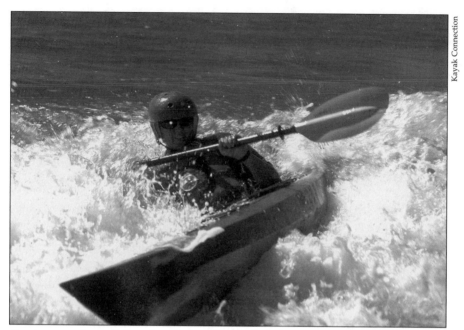

Kayakers can always find good surfing conditions along this coast

Continuing down the coast you have to go well offshore to get around the kelp beds before you reach the Capitola Wharf. You are now 3.5 miles northeast along the coast from Santa Cruz Harbor. There is a handy, little sand beach where you can land on the near side of the wharf. It is the beginning of Capitola Beach, most of which is the other side of the wharf. As you leave Capitola Beach behind, there is an outcrop of rocks with a little cove behind it and a small surf running into the cove. It is an ideal spot for kayak-surfing beginners. As you look down the sweeping curve of the coast, the old shipwreck off Seacliff State Beach comes into view. When you get there, you have come 5 miles. It's a long, long beach that continues southeast to Elkhorn Slough, 15 miles away.

Typically, the sea off Santa Cruz is extremely calm in the early morning, when flat-water scullers take their rigs out to sea. By late morning there is always some wave action, and by mid-afternoon it can get quite choppy out there. Since you will probably be paddling into the wind on the way back to Santa Cruz, allow plenty of time for your return. The Kayak Connection runs guided trips down to the otters' territory, but if you do it alone and find yourself unable to make a safe return, you can land at well-sheltered Capitola Beach and give the Kayak Connection a call (415) 479-1121. For a small fee, they will drive there and taxi you and your kayak to your car.

◄── ≡◆≡ ──►

In the major kelp plantation off Soquel and Pleasure points sea otters breed and raise their young. They lie on their backs to eat and use their chests as platforms, not only for the anvil rocks on which they break open their food, but to carry their nursing and napping young. Obviously, when you see this happening, stay well away from them and use your binoculars, rather than crowding to get a camera shot. When they are really curious, they will stand up in the water—with almost half their bodies clear of it—and may appear to clap hands as though applauding you. They are about 30 inches long, and are a furry wet-brown all over. The older males develop white heads and look quite distinguished as they go about their business of feeding, and also watching you watch them.

Sea otters usually have only one offspring at a time. These are born at sea in the spring, with their eyes open and fur and teeth all ready to go. It takes the mothers a full year to wean their young, though the young may remain around their mothers longer. Sometimes you will see otters so ensnared in kelp that you may think they are trapped, but they are not. They like to dress up in kelp and, by doing so, moor themselves so that neither wind nor tide can dislodge them. The largest number of sea otters I have had in sight at one time was in the huge kelp bed off Pleasure Point. There were 47 adult sea otters at the surface, and there must have been more down below.

Once when I was out well beyond the Santa Cruz 1-mile buoy, planning a fast run back to the harbor pushed by a strong wind and a following sea, I made a unique kayak connection. But not with otters. I had just turned about and was looking for the harbor entrance when I saw several dark birds approaching me. They were not close together and looked awkward in flight as they came low over the water. In fact, their approach was so erratic that for a while I wasn't sure they knew what they were doing. They were dark enough to be young Heermann's gulls, but they didn't fly like any gull. They even looked as though they might fall into the water. And then I realized they were sooty shearwaters. They were not gliding in troughs between the waves as they usually do, like skiers cruising around moguls. They were almost bumping over the mogul-like waves to get to me.

One landed right beside me—very clumsily and not at all gull-like—then another and another. Soon there were seven in front of my cockpit, on either side, and all were tapping with their beaks on the hull of my black Arluk II—the stealth boat. With a lot of movement in the water, they were tossed around while still tapping. I was astounded by what was happening, even as I took in the details of their specialized beaks which I'd never seen this close before. I could see why these birds, from the middle group of the albatross family (the shearwaters), are called tubinars: *two tubes raised on either side of their upper mandibles have the specific function of discharging excess salt solution, accumulating from their pelagic feeding habits.*

So here we were: one kayaker sitting upright in an all-black, 18-foot kayak; and a small group of hungry, sooty shearwaters that had probably mistaken me for a black, basking shark, and were hoping to nibble a few tidbits off my skin. I sat there, with my body sized and placed similarly to a basking shark's dorsal fin when lying surfaced. My kayak was about the right length, too. How do I make this connection? Because, as Walt Whitman said, "The unseen is proved by the seen." And, like the shearwaters, I carry that with me wherever I go. Usually, it works for me just fine.

Wildlife of California's Central Coast

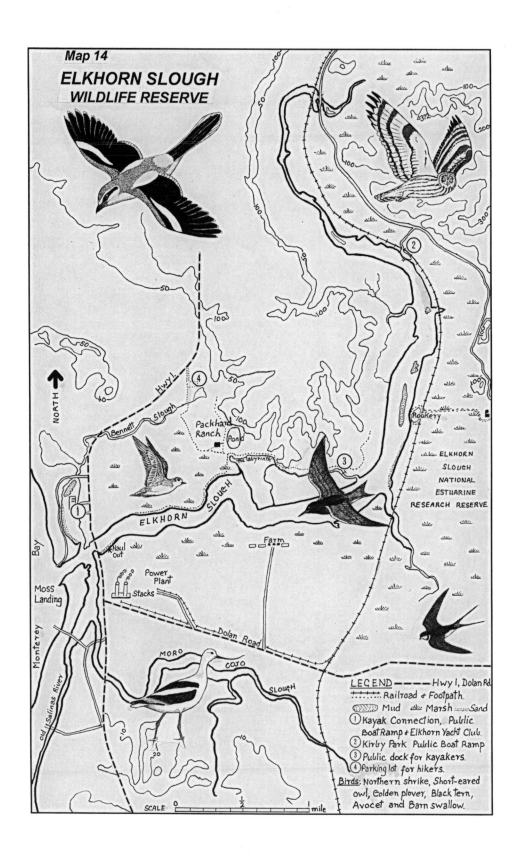

Map 14
ELKHORN SLOUGH
WILDLIFE RESERVE

NORTH

Hwy 1

Bennett Slough

Packhard Ranch

Pond

The Labyrinth

ELKHORN SLOUGH

Rookery

ELKHORN
SLOUGH
NATIONAL
ESTUARINE
RESEARCH RESERVE

Bay

Haul Out

Moss Landing

Monterey

Power Plant

Stacks

Farm

Dolan Road

MORO

COJO

SLOUGH

Old Salinas River

LEGEND ———— Hwy 1, Dolan Rd
:::::::: Railroad & Footpath.
Mud   Marsh Sand
① Kayak Connection, Public
    Boat Ramp & Elkhorn Yacht Club.
② Kirby Park Public Boat Ramp
③ Public dock for kayakers.
④ Parking lot for hikers.
Birds: Northern shrike, Short-eared
owl, Golden plover, Black Tern,
Avocet and Barn swallow.

SCALE 0   ½   1 mile

TRIP 18 ELKHORN SLOUGH:
Kirby Park to Moss Landing

Type	Length	Map
Moderate full day	10 miles RT to Moss Landing	14
Easy half-day shuttle	5 miles one way to Moss Landing	14
Easy half day	4 miles RT to railroad trestle	14

Summary and Highlights

Elkhorn Slough is one of California's best marine life sanctuaries and bird-watching venues. The mouth of the slough is at Moss Landing, halfway between Santa Cruz and Monterey, and the slough's broad waterway winds for 7 miles into the strawberry-growing hinterland. For kayaking purposes there are two public access areas: the public boat ramp at Moss Landing, and the public boat dock, 5 miles inland at Kirby Park. For a one-way trip you can shuttle between these points. The Kayak Connection has an on-water facility at the Elkhorn Yacht Club near Moss Landing (408) 724-5692. They offer rentals, sales, instruction, and guided tours, starting and ending at the yacht club harbor. The Kirby Park put-in point has plenty of free parking and is much less crowded on weekends than Moss Landing. It is also better for kayaking novices on their own, and for canoeists, because it is more sheltered.

The countryside for the entire 7 miles along the north shore is hilly, grassy, and unspoiled. We owe its preservation to the Packard Foundation and the Elkhorn Slough Foundation, under management and protection of the California Department of Fish and Game. A good walking trail along the slough's north side is maintained, but the outstanding wildlife of the slough cannot be seen better than by kayak.

Special Advice

The prevailing wind on the slough is from the ocean, and it can get very strong in the afternoons. Two giant stacks emitting steam from the Dolan Industrial Park are excellent indicators for what the wind is up to. Having to slog into a headwind returning to Moss Landing should be factored into your day's trip. Perhaps only in the US can you find this next anomaly. Elkhorn Slough is a marine mammal and bird sanctuary, with a pistol range on its south shore between it and the industrial chimneys. You'll be relieved to know that it is illegal to fire any weapon over navigable water. Another anomaly is that Elkhorn Slough is a duck-hunting venue as well as a bird sanctuary. In the winter months, don't be surprised to see a dozen, khaki-clad figures lining the north bank—men and a few women—with their 12-gauge shotguns. They are waiting for the ducks they can't shoot over the Packard Ranch; these are ducks that come and go to a particularly nutritious and tranquil pond out of public sight. By law, the hunters should at no time be firing over any kayaker's head, but they may aim the other way. And the duck that is hit may well crash into the pickleweed or water around you. Very strange!

How to Get There

Coming from the south, to put in at Moss Landing, which is 25 miles north of Monterey, take Route 1. As you approach Moss Landing, you will see the twin chimney stacks of Dolan Industrial Park ahead of you for many miles. When you reach them, you'll have only 0.8 mile to go. Right after passing the industrial park, you cross over Elkhorn Slough. The Elkhorn Yacht Club is on the left side of the highway 0.7 mile beyond the bridge. There is a large earthen-ware pottery business and a narrow, paved entrance to the public boating access on the left, in front of the yacht club. And, 60 yards beyond the boating access is the entrance to the yacht club and the Kayak Connection.

Coming from the north: The Elkhorn Yacht Club is 25 miles south of Santa Cruz, on Route 1. When the Dolan Industrial Park twin chimneys are in plain sight, look for the pottery business and numerous small yachts in front of the yacht club, on your right. The first entrance is to the yacht club and the Kayak Connection; the second entrance, 60 yards farther, is to the public boating access. If you use the public boat ramp and dock, there is a $5 charge. There are lavatory facilities on site. If you park on the open space south of the parking lot and put in from any of the small sand beaches in the area, there is no charge. This is where to leave a car if you intend to make a one-way trip from Kirby Park to Moss Landing.

For the inland, Kirby Park Public Access: coming from the south on Route 1, turn right onto Dolan Rd. (later Castro Blvd.), in front of the Dolan Industrial Park. In 3.5 miles, turn left onto Elkhorn Rd. The entrance to Elkhorn Slough National Estuarine Research Reserve will be on your left in another 2 miles. The visitor center is well worth checking into for information, local maps, and guide books. In another 2.5 miles the entrance to Kirby Park Public Access is on your left. Turn left, and go 0.25 mile to the railroad crossing stop sign. Cross the tracks and head left to the far end of the long parking lot. You will find the boat dock on your right.

Coming from the north on Route 1 for Kirby Park, go 14.6 miles south of Santa Cruz and turn left at a hilltop onto Salinas Rd. There is a small store and gas station 0.8 mile down Salinas Rd., and a public golf course. 15.8 miles from Santa Cruz, turn right on Werner Rd. At 16 miles, turn right onto

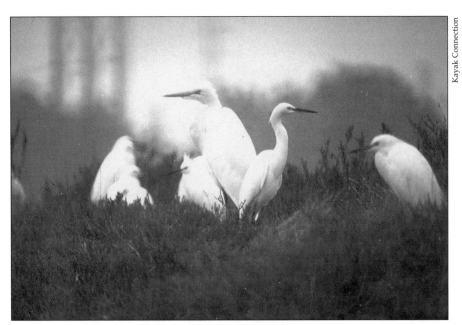

Intimate views of snowy and great egrets along the slough

Elkhorn Rd. At 16.8 miles, turn right for Elkhorn Slough. At 17.7 miles, a roadrail trestle over the slough is on your right, and this trestle is as far as you can paddle inland. Turn right at the sign for Kirby Park Public Access, after 19 miles.

Trip Description

Exploring Elkhorn Slough from Kirby Park is preferable because of easier parking and less scrambling to get on the water—especially when it's open salmon season. Then, the Moss Landing public parking lot is packed, the harbor channel to the dock is crowded with boats, and nauseous engine fumes fill the air. The Moss Landing area is fine out of season, but the sun is in the right place for the entire day from the Kirby Park put-in point. The wind, too, is usually favorable in the afternoon for the return to Kirby Park. It's up to you to pick a day when the tides favor you—both coming and going.

One option from Kirby Park is to turn right from the jetty and paddle 2 miles farther inland, stopping where the railroad tracks cross the slough. You see plenty of egrets, herons, and some shorebirds this way; but you are unlikely to find sea otters because the water's too shallow. It's a good direction to take if you are inexperienced, on your own, and want a safe route. It's also a good way to go if you've come to the slough and the wind feels too strong for you to head toward the ocean.

The ocean is 5 miles away, going left from the jetty, and there are only two good haul-out spots before the Route 1 bridge. The first is a kayak dock 2 miles away on the right side; the second is 4.75 miles to a pleasant sand beach on your left just before the bridge. After the bridge, the best haul-out place is another 0.25 mile to the right side of the rip-rap at the estuary's mouth.

Heading 0.25 mile toward the ocean from Kirby Park, you'll see on your right a small posted sign naming the wildlife reserve. There may be a small Forster's tern sitting on it. Behind this sign are many acres of mud at low tide. Paddle toward this marker when you see it, and leave it on your right as you go. In 1 mile, on the right, you'll see a fairly broad channel cutting into the mud and pickleweed, that stretches for a half mile to the grassland and trees bordering the slough's north side. You can follow this channel to that border. It's fun, but you won't see nearly as much of the marsh or as many shorebirds as you will by staying in the mainstream.

Close to the east shore, opposite this channel entrance, there is a muddy island. A half mile farther, a grove of eucalyptus trees close to the shore has an egrets' rookery in its lofty shelter. All this land is in the care of the Elkhorn Slough Estuarine Research Reserve. If you stay on this side of the slough it will curve around to the south, bringing you to the railroad tracks you crossed earlier at Kirby Park. Behind the train trestle is a vast area of marsh, strictly off limits. But by gliding among the supporting trestle timbers, you can at least take a peek at where you're not allowed to go. This off-limits area

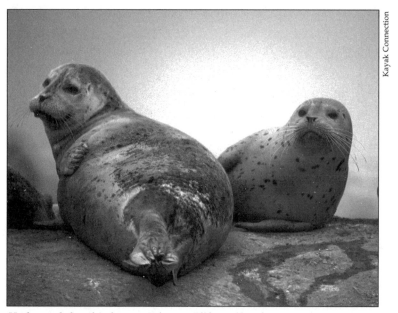

Harbor seals breed in large numbers at Elkhorn Slough

is an important breeding sanctuary for elegant terns, summer visitors that haven't been doing too well recently, for reasons not yet confirmed. There may not be enough fish of the right size in the slough to support a large colony of terns.

On the north shore, 2 miles from Kirby Park there is a broad channel going off to your right. You can see a bench on high, open ground in front of you, and to the left there is a lovely grove of old black oaks. You can enter this channel on any tide to reach the wooden steps and small dock put in specifically for kayakers by the California Conservation Corps. If you stop here for a break, make sure you line your boat off the dock. (Your kayak should have a bow line long enough for a number of situations, including towing another kayaker, or floating your kayak off a dock so that other people can come alongside, too.) There are two toilets discreetly placed just off the trail under the trees. That trail leads from the oak grove onto high ground where there is the bench that you saw from your kayak that offers a fine overview of the slough.

If there's a reasonably high tide (above 5 feet), you can stay in this channel and paddle the whole length of "the labyrinth" until it rejoins the main slough in a mile. If you do you'll be paddling beside the trail that borders the slough. About halfway along the labyrinth there is another channel to the left that heads back into the slough. You can take this or, if there's enough water, keep going to complete the labyrinth. If you do this, there is a single-strand barbed wire fence in the pickleweed between you and the trail and, to continue, you will probably have to go under this wire into a diversionary channel. You must negotiate about 40 yards of what is really a ditch and—turning left under the same wire—get back into the channel.

Now, with plenty of water, the narrow channel swings left into a long, straight line of water. Follow this channel, and when it starts winding again, stay with the main flow. Except for the few minutes when the tide peaks (and when it bottoms out), there will be a visible direction of flow in this channel. When you come out into the broadwater of the slough, you'll be 1.25 miles from the Route 1 bridge. You can't see it because there's a big bend ahead, but you can hear the tractor trailers roaring along the highway. You are now in sea otter territory, and there are many of them from here to Moss Landing. As you take the last bend in the slough before the bridge, there is a major seal haul out behind a broken down bank on your right. Do not bother these seals; they breed here and panic easily. As you round this last bend, the mud bank is in good repair and is quite high. It's a favorite drying-out spot for pelicans and cormorants. Enjoy them, but give them plenty of room so as not to disturb them.

If, after landing at the kayakers' dock, or bypassing the labyrinth, you continued toward Moss Landing on the mainstream, you'd be heading into the windy section of the slough. The water doesn't get rough, but the wind can blow. If you find yourself against it, follow the south shore to the bridge. For the next 1.5 miles, it will be more sheltered on that side. But when it's not too windy, mid-stream is a good place to meet sea otters. They are very calm in this area, and you can hear them banging clams on their chest-held rock anvils, even when you can't see them.

By the time you reach the main U-bend, where the otter colony hangs out, you will be 4 miles from Kirby Park. The second haul-out spot for this trip is the beach on the left, before the bridge. If you are continuing under the bridge, whether the tide is going in or out, but particularly if it's pouring out to sea, aim for the bridge's right-hand corner. If you are nicely lined up, you'll have no difficulty in turning right, in spite of a very powerful current, into the harbor. If there are standing, bouncing waves under the bridge, lucky you. Point your kayak straight into the flow and go for it. If you want to haul out on the little sand beach just inside the entrance to the harbor, it's visible to the right of the riprap and only 200 yards away.

⊷ ⊱◆⊰ ⊶

Mark Pastick, of the Kayak Connection, calls me "the Warden of Elkhorn Slough," and I wish I were because the slough is a national treasure that is readily abused. Chemicals from intensive strawberry cultivation on the surrounding hills stream into the slough with every rainfall; recreational boaters (not anglers) come tearing through the slough with wakes that rip into the fragile mud banks; and hunters wing waterfowl that are irretrievable because of the private and public multi-use claims on this land. The hunters know the rules, and from what I've seen they follow them. It's just that the ducks don't know which side of the fence to come down on when they're hit. I'm not against duck hunting. But there are so many users and abusers on the slough. Some would say there are too many kayakers, and they might be right, given that there is always a conflict of interests in the use of a designated "multiple use" area.

As a kayaker paddling Elkhorn Slough, you are likely to see a quiet pontoon boat gliding through on a guided tour. It's skippered by Captain Yohn Gideon, often accompanied by his naturalist wife, Melanie. From this very stable observation platform they lead birdwatching trips specializing in shorebirds, and explaining the history and ecology of the slough. This is an ideal option for those who don't want to, or can't, go kayaking, and for elderly people. The boarding point for these trips is at Moss Landing Fishing Boat Harbor, on the south side of the bridge over Elkhorn Slough. The trips last approximately two hours. Call (408) 633-5555 for schedules and reservations.

Elkhorn Slough provides room to roam for a whole day's bird watching without running out of navigable water. I know where all the different species like to hang out, and what's likely to be around at any time of year. In spring, late summer, and fall, the slough is outstanding for shorebirds in great numbers and variety. As you glide along with the current, you can smoothly plug the bow of your kayak into the oozing banks and watch many species of sandpipers, so close to you that you don't need binoculars. They are not worried by kayakers; they are too busy probing the mud for food. The rarer sandpipers that I've seen in the past two years are a stilt sandpiper, a red phalarope, a golden plover (really golden), a Wilson's plover, pectoral sandpipers, and a rufous-necked stint.

In the air, or standing on the banks, Caspian and elegant terns appear throughout the summer, and the Forster's tern is here year round. I've also seen the rare common tern (common on the East Coast) and the endangered least tern, only 9 inches long. And in 1997, a superb black tern in full summer plumage was also seen. I had seven clients with me the day we saw the black tern. We watched it hawking for insects rather than fish as all the other terns do, and it was more agile in the air than any other in its family. If ever terns deserved to be known as "sea swallows" as they are, this tern should take the credit. It landed on the mud and stood beside a Caspian tern, more than twice its length and twice its wingspan; a David with Goliath, among terns. It was the most beautiful bird I've seen in 15 years on the slough: it's head and body were jet black, fading to a gray rump and tail. The upper surface of its wings was the same gray, but the under surface was a lighter gray. All its lower body was purely white, contrasting brilliantly in the bright sunlight with the blackness of its belly. We were able to glide within two kayak lengths from the black tern before it decided to continue its aerial ballet. And its incredible agility in flight fascinated us; it was the Barishnikov of all the birds on the wing.

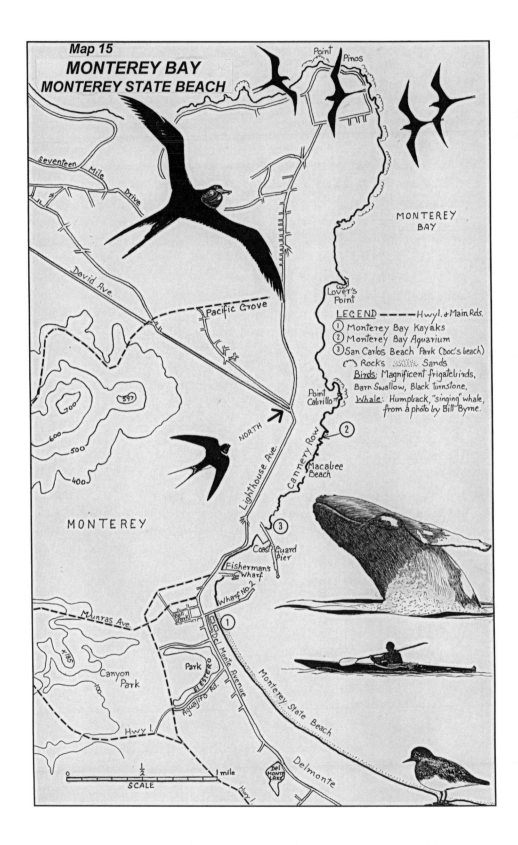

Map 15
MONTEREY BAY
MONTEREY STATE BEACH

Point
Pinos

seventeen Mile Drive

MONTEREY BAY

David Ave.

Pacific Grove

Lover's Point

LEGEND ———— Hwyl. & Main Rds.
① Monterey Bay Kayaks
② Monterey Bay Aquarium
③ San Carlos Beach Park (Doc's beach)
Rocks   Sands
Birds: Magnificent frigatebirds,
Barn Swallow, Black turnstone,
Whale: Humpback, "singing" whale,
from a photo by Bill Byrne.

597

700

600

500

400

NORTH

Point Cabrillo

②

Lighthouse Ave.

Cannery Row

Macabee Beach

MONTEREY

③

Coast Guard Pier

Fisherman's Wharf

Wharf No. 2

Munras Ave.

①

185

Canyon Park

Park

Del Monte Avenue

EL ESTERO

Aguajito Rd.

Hwy 1

Monterey State Beach

Delmonte

0   ½   1 mile
SCALE

Del Monte Lake

Hwy 1

TRIP 19 MONTEREY'S WATERFRONT

Type	Length	Map
Easy half-day exploring	3–6 miles RT	15

Summary and Highlights

Monterey Bay, named in 1602 for the Count of Monte Rey, was sighted 60 years earlier by Juan Rodriguez Cabrillo. The Monterey Peninsula, with Pacific Grove—famous for its wintering monarch butter-flies—on its northern shore, shields the southern corner of Monterey Bay. You'll find Monterey Bay Kayaks (MBK) there, with a perfect waterfront for putting in on the bay. They use a public beach with limited public parking at its entrance next to MBK. Cass and Jeff Shrock, the owners of MBK, welcome independent kayakers to use their facility. Park with them during the week, but you must find your own parking on weekends and holidays. Their store features an outstanding variety of kayaks and all accessories, plus a good book section, complete with maps. They offer rentals, lessons, guided tours, and advanced paddling-technique clinics with two of the West Coast's best, offshore-distance racers, Brent Reitz and Mike McNulty. For further information call (408) 373-5357.

A kayak trip in the southern corner of the bay is remarkable for the variety of marine life. There are sea otters, sea lions, and harbor seals in great numbers. Young northern elephant seals, wandering down from the major breeding ground for these largest of all pinnipeds, put in an appearance. They come from Año Nuevo, 85 miles to the north. Whales—mostly big grays—migrating down the coast are often visible offshore from a kayak.

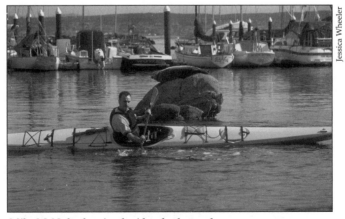

Mike McNulty bracing beside a harbor seal

Special Advice

There are two things to remember. One is that the calmness in this southern corner of the bay, in front of MBK, does not guarantee calmness once you are clear of the harboring wharves and piers. Don't paddle beyond Point Cabrillo, on the north shore of the peninsula, unless you are prepared to meet some very big swells—I mean 30-foot swells, or greater. Unless you are sure of your solo-paddling competence, the best thing to do is join a guided tour or take a lesson with MBK.

The other thing concerns protection of the marine mammals in the bay; some are so absurdly tame that you can't avoid them, while others are extremely nervous. There are two rules you should follow in approaching them (they are rules, not just guidelines). First, no matter how far you are away from them, whenever you are approaching seals, otters, or any other species, if you see them getting ready to avoid you, or already doing so, either change direction or backoff. Second, never feed them, however tame and friendly any of these wild creatures appear to be.

How to Get There

From north of Monterey, take Route 1 south. The Fort Ord ex-Military Reservation, which is now a college campus, is on your left as you approach Monterey, and there are sweeping views of the bay on your right. Take the PACIFIC GROVE—DEL MONTE AVE exit. Follow Del Monte Ave. for 1.45 miles, turning right at the first light and left at the ocean front. Public parking is on your right, in front of Monterey Bay Kayaks at 693 Del Monte Ave.

From Salinas: Follow Route 68 west to Monterey. Take Route 1 south, and stay in the right lane. Take the DOWNTOWN MONTEREY exit, and turn right at the first light on Camino Aguajito. Turn left on Del Monte Ave., and follow it to MBK, at 693 Del Monte Ave.

From south of Monterey: Follow Route 1 north to Monterey, and take the AGUAJITO RD. exit. Turn left on Aguajito and left at Del Monte Ave. MBK is on your right at 693 Del Monte Ave.

Trip Description

This trip goes only 3 miles from your put-in point in front of Monterey Bay Kayaks. It is a safe exploration trip for the beginner and a satisfying experience for the expert paddler, too, because there is so much to see, both historically and ecologically, from your kayak. Everything is amazingly accessible. As you put in from Monterey State Beach, right in front of MBK, you'll be facing north. There will be a few yachts at anchor; the water will be calm, with probably only a one-foot wavelet breaking on the beach. To your left there's the almost half-mile long, Municipal Wharf No.2 pointing north, and you will head north to get around it. It bends to the west and, if you look shoreward, at the end of it

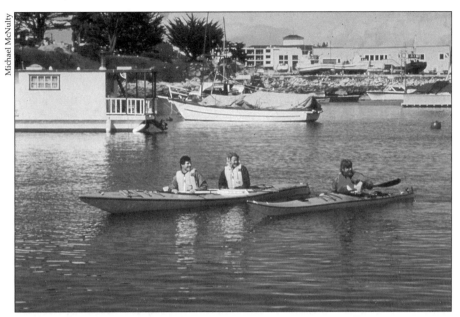

Michael McNulty

You can see a wide variety of birds, pinnipeds, as well as historical sites along Monterey's waterfront

you'll see Monterey Marina and Fisherman's Wharf. Beyond that is the long, Coast Guard Pier, that comes out from the shore and heads east.

The long arms of Wharf No.2 and Coast Guard Pier, known as "the Breakwater," protect the marina, which is the hub of a great deal of marine activity. In this sheltered area there are two boat ramps, many slips and moorings, and boat rentals. Fisherman's Wharf, which juts out into the Marina, is host to fish markets, fishing trips, and sight-seeing cruises of the bay, as well as open-sea trips for whale watching and bird watching. All of this activity is fascinating to watch from a kayak, but you must keep alert and out of the way.

Paddling beyond the Coast Guard Pier, you will be offshore from San Carlos Beach and one of the English-speaking world's great literary landmarks, Cannery Row. A great sardine-canning industry flourished here for 50 years until 1951 when the sardines vanished from Monterey Bay. And it was from here that John Steinbeck sent his fictional alter ego, the marine biologist "Doc," to the tidepools along San Carlos Beach to collect specimens for marine labs.

As you circumvent the wonderful rock formations that turn this part of the coast into a dramatic rock park, paddling toward the sandy cove of Macabee Beach, you will almost certainly meet individual divers or diving classes in this area. Unlike Doc's commercial collecting, these divers' efforts will be strictly recreational because no marine life may be removed from the Monterey Bay Sanctuary, except by permit for scientific research.

The next, interesting shoreline feature from your sea-level vantage is that remarkable achievement, the Monterey Bay Aquarium. It's built on the old, Hovden Cannery site and houses living, in- and outdoor exhibits of everything living in the bay. It is a marvelous thing to see what you can see paddling in the bay, and later visit the aquarium to find out a great deal more about what it is you have seen. (The Monterey Bay Aquarium is open every day of the year, except Christmas Day, from 10 A.M.-6 P.M. For more information, call (800) 840-4880.)

All throughout this trip you'll meet sea otters, harbor seals, sea lions, and other kayakers. You'll encounter pelicans, cormorants, scoters, loons, and grebes diving for fish, or cruising around (as you are). All sorts of crustaceans thrive on the rocky ledges and outcrops that are constantly scrubbed by the wave action, and also treated to the air and sun by alternate periods of tidal submersion and exposure. Some are attached to the rocks while others are mobile, but in either case there are several birds that specialize in harvesting them. And they are easy to identify.

There are, of course, omnivorous gulls constantly surveying the scene and chipping away at those items on their menu attached to the rocks (muscles, whelks, and barnacles) and snatching crabs and anything else edible. Their name, *gullo*, in Latin means "greedy." The specialists, though, are shorebirds: the black oystercatcher—with its big black-brown body and brilliant-red beak; the wandering tattler—like a smaller willet, but with no black and white in its wings when it flies; black turnstones—small, black-and-white birds, always chittering and running; and the whimbrel. The first three of these work along the waterline, constantly moving from one outcrop of rocks to the next, and often getting drenched by water breaking on the rocks. But the whimbrel, with its long down-curved beak, looks like a small long-billed curlew, and it stays a little higher and dryer on the rocks.

━━ ≣◆≣ ━━

In 1993, I taught English literature at a high school in Monterey, covering for someone on a sabbatical leave. My 12 seniors, most of them without much interest in studying English, were ideal candidates for an excursion outside their curriculum. We needed a motivational tool for them to take advantage of their school's interest in educating them. So I took them down to Monterey Bay Kayaks for an afternoon-evening session on the water, with an agreement that each one of them would write an essay about the experience.

None of the seniors had ever been kayaking, and only two had ever worn a wetsuit. Since MBKs safety requirements include keeping its clientele warm, they suited up and seized their paddles as if getting ready for a jousting tournament. We went down to the beach where an MBK staff member took them through their paddle-handling drills. Their flair for participation on the water wasn't looking much better than in the classroom. There were questions like: "How long are we going to be out here?" "Why do I have to be in the same boat as Melanie?" "Will we get back before dark?" "Where are we going?"

I hoped my answer to the last question would be good enough to finally get these kids' attention. "We are on our way to meet a whale!" And that got their attention. An adult gray whale had been living in the bay for several weeks, and unless it had made its move overnight, I expected it to be somewhere between Fisherman's Wharf and Monterey Bay Aquarium, where I had seen it the previous day. This enormous creature was at the time living under, or unwillingly carrying, an enormous canopy of kelp. While it wasn't going to be as dramatic as a whale at sea, as long as it moved it would still be impressive. If it didn't move, I knew I was in trouble; if it didn't move we were unlikely to find it.

The search was on, and with frequent reinforcement curiosity was running at a high peak. After an hour or more went by, we'd gone well beyond the place where I'd seen the whale. At least, I'd seen the shape of its rounded back and a huge mound of moving kelp. I was regretting my idea and feeling discouraged when there was an extraordinary movement in the kelp just ahead of us. The kelp canopy in front of us was rising like dough in an oven: rising in very slow motion, but rising higher and higher while moving forward. Then, just as slowly, it was subsiding. We all stopped and waited, needing confirmation that what we thought we'd seen wasn't an illusion.

We waited patiently. And we nearly missed the whale because, though the kelp was rising again, it was far ahead of where we'd seen it the first time. We paddled, trying to close the gap between us until we saw its rising bulk once more, still going away from us. It seemed to be heading out to sea, taking its canopy with it, and it was time for us to turn back. The students all wrote their essays, and some in the class swore they had seen the whale's black back. On one point all concurred—it was a "really cool" experience.

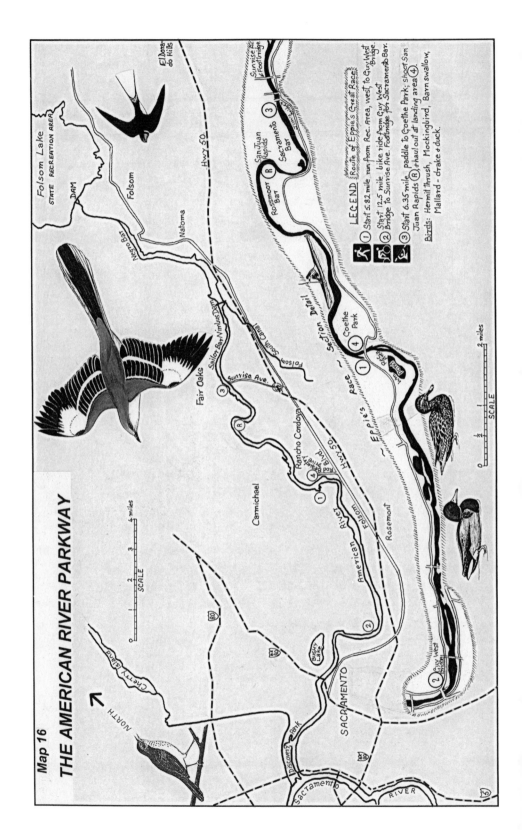

Map 16
THE AMERICAN RIVER PARKWAY

Folsom Lake
STATE RECREATION AREA

El Dorado Hills

Folsom
DAM

Negro Bar

Nimbus Dam
Sailor Bar

Natoma

Hwy 50

Fair Oaks

Sunrise Ave.
3

Folsom South Canal

Rosmoor Bar

San Juan Rapids
R

Sacramento Bar

Sunrise Fwy. Footbridge
3

Section Detail

Rancho Cordova

Red Bridge
R
4
1

Hwy 50

Eppie's Race

Goethe Park
4
1

Carmichael

American River

Folsom River

Rosemont

SCALE
0   1   2   3   4 miles

NORTH

Cherry Island

Discovery Park

Sacramento River

SACRAMENTO

Bushy Lake

Guy West Bridge
2

80

50

99

SCALE
0   ½   1   2 miles

LEGEND
Route of Eppie's Great Race
① Start 5.82 mile run from Rec. Area, west, to Guy West Bridge.
② Start 12.5 mile bike ride from Guy West Bridge to Sunrise Ave. Footbridge for Sacramento Bar.
③ Start 6.35 mile paddle to Goethe Park; shoot San Juan Rapids ℝ; haul out at landing area ④.
Birds: Hermit Thrush, Mockingbird, Barn swallow, Mallard - drake & duck.

Chapter 10

Sacramento

TRIP 20 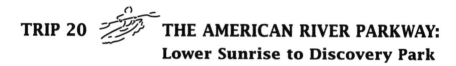 **THE AMERICAN RIVER PARKWAY:**
Lower Sunrise to Discovery Park

Type	Length	Map
Full-day shuttle	20 miles one way	16
Strenuous half day (if done as part of triathlon race)	6.35 miles one way to Goethe Park	16
Easy half-day shuttle	6.35 miles one way to Goethe Park	16

Summary and Highlights

Eppie Johnson, kayaker and restaurateur, and one of the nation's "citizen athletes" chosen to be a torch bearer in the 1996 Olympic Torch Relay to Atlanta, claims the triathlon race he started 25 years ago has the longest history of any such event in the world. Eppie's "Great Race" takes place along the bike path beside the American River and on the river itself. It is a showcase for the kayak-canoe potential of the American River Parkway. Eppie's race starts 15 miles east of Sacramento, in the Rancho Cordova area of the American River. The event is held in July when more than 1,000 paddlers race a little over 6 miles down the swiftly flowing river. Through this remarkable riparian environment they compete, boat to boat, in the wildest variety of kayaks and canoes. This is the last leg of the 5.82-mile run, 12.5-mile bike, and 6.35-mile down-river paddle, that adds up to a 24.67-mile, triathlon adventure.

You can enter this event as a team member or go the "iron person" route and do it all. The kayaking component is exciting, but safe for a novice paddler. The one technical rapid on the course is an easy Class 3, closely monitored for safety during the race so that beginners can definitely go for it. Helmets, foot protection, and life jackets are mandatory. California Canoe & Kayak (CCK), with John Stofer managing (916) 631-1400, have their river canoe-kayak rentals, sales, and teaching program situated by the American River, right where Eppie's downriver event starts. They share their site with American River Raft Rentals (916) 635-6400. Both companies offer helpful advice to independent paddlers who may want to explore all 20 miles from their Lower Sunrise site, downstream to the American River's confluence with the Sacramento River. To do this a shuttle vehicle can be left at Discovery Park.

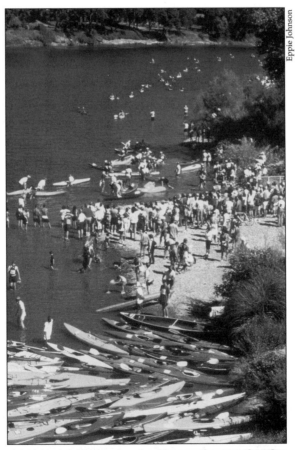

As many as 1,000 kayakers land here as they complete the last leg of Eppie's Great Race

Special Advice

The American River Parkway is used commercially by rafting and paddling companies from mid-April to mid-October, and this should be your
timeframe for use of it, if you are inexperienced. Dan Crandall and Colleen
McKinnon of Current Adventures Kayaking (916) 642-9755, will give expert
advice or kayaking instruction for those needing it on the river. In conjunc-
tion with River City Paddlers, Inc., they offer a warm-up paddle race, guid-
ing newcomers through the actual course of the kayaking event in Eppie's
Great Race.

The main threat to any boater on this river is submerged tree snags, particularly around the pillars supporting bridges. Aim for the middle of a span
as you pass under bridges. Daily river flow rates are available by calling the
Bureau of Reclamation at (916) 979-2330, ext. 102.

How to Get There

From the Bay Area: for the California Canoe & Kayak put-in point and the
Lower Sunrise Public Access, head east on Interstate 80. Just before
Sacramento take the Highway 50 exit for SOUTH LAKE TAHOE & SACRAMENTO. In
3 miles you cross the Sacramento River and continue on Highway 50, now
following the SOUTH LAKE TAHOE & PLACERVILLE sign. In 19 miles a big sign
announces the American River Sunrise Exit, well before the exit. In 1 mile
take the SUNRISE EXIT north onto Sunrise Blvd. Continue 1.3 miles north to
South Bridge St. As you turn right, CCK and American River Raft Rentals are
in front of you. For public access to the river, continue on South Bridge St.
past CCK for 0.35 mile to the American River Parkway's kiosk. Pay $4 for day
parking in the Lower Sunrise River Access lot, and $2 for boat launching. It's
open 5 A.M.-10 P.M. throughout the summer.

Trip Description

There are 20 miles open for paddling, swimming, fishing, and picnicking
on the American River Parkway along the river's fast-flowing westward
course. The first few miles at the parkway's east end above the Nimbus Dam
are not available for putting in because that part of the river, called Lake
Natoma, is a second reservoir. It serves as the regulator for the Folsom Dam,
feeding water to the San Joaquin Valley. The best point of entry to the river is
below Sailor Bar (a gravel bar), though you could put in at the bar. It's tempting to do so, if only to get the most mileage out of your riparian, parkland
paddle. But your best put-in point is at Lower Sunrise River Access, opposite
the Sacramento Bar, where the kayak event starts in Eppie's Great Race.

Even in midsummer, the water flows at a swift 2+ mph, and it takes little
time to cover the 6.35 miles down to C.M. Goethe Park, where Eppie's race
ends. You could float down there in two to three hours, and certainly paddle

it in little more than an hour. But there's much to enjoy, and on a full day trip you can continue safely all the way to Discovery or Goethe Parks, 20 miles downstream from Lower Sunrise. Or you can take out at several other parks on your way west. Ask at CCK or the American River Raft Rentals for directions to Discovery or Goethe Parks to leave your shuttle vehicle there, or for shuttle service they sometimes provide to Discovery Park, Goethe Park, or other haul-out points.

The land for Goethe (pronounced "gay-tee") Park was donated by that family. It is a splendid picnic area shaded by many large oak trees, and home to deer and wild turkeys in the quiet hours. The entire parkway is a green recreation ribbon, most remarkable for its proximity to the gray world of commerce.

Continuing 2 miles downstream from Goethe Park you come to Arden Bar and the William B. Pond Recreation Area, where you can take out. The next picnic area is 3.5 miles farther, by the Watt Ave. Bridge. In another 4 miles you come to the park at Bushy Lake, where the exotic, surface-feeding wood duck nests in tree holes well above ground. Anywhere, all spring and summer, you are going to meet the American merganser on the river; this handsome diving bird's presence signals fishing. And you'll see kayakers and rafters indolently drifting downstream, trolling for stripers and salmon. You'll certainly spot red-tailed hawks and a few white-tailed kites that look as weightless as wind-blown paper, quartering the ground for mice.

You come to Discovery Park at Bannon Slough in another 4 miles downstream. Your route ends here, unless you are heading south, in which case you could go all the way to San Francisco. Along this entire route there is a

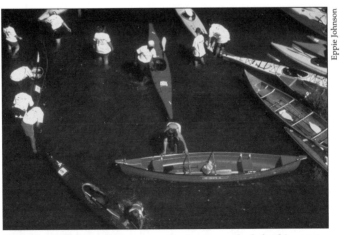

Racers pass their kayaks to scores of volunteers who help this event run smoothly

great variety of wildlife. Chinook salmon, steelhead, shad, striped bass, and two Sacramento specialties—squawfish and sucker—are found in the American River. There are river otters and beavers; and mountain lions may pass through the parkway, if only traversing this section of riparian corridor that leads from the Central valley to the Sierra Nevada.

There is an excellent map of the American River Parkway, obtainable for $3 at CCK on the river, or by mail from The American River Parkway Foundation at P.O. Box 188437, Sacramento, CA 95818 (916) 456-7423. It describes the flora and fauna of the parkway with text and good illustrations. It also shows in detail all the roads leading to the many picnic areas and possible put-in points.

Logistics, keeping track of your gear, and knowing the ground rules whenever you are in a populated outdoor recreational area: these are three cardinal points that, if not attended to, can turn a trip into a near misadventure. Mass starts in adventure racing are a spawning ground for such happenings. When I competed in the "iron person" class of Eppie's Great Race, I had no knowledge of the area at all. Though the rules were clear, and the race organization was impeccable, it was hard to comply for my sheer lack of preparation for the event. Personal organization and at least one helper are a must for participation in the "iron" division.

Keith Kiellor, designer of the Valhalla surf ski, brought me one from San Diego for the race, and dropped it off with his own surf ski on the Sacramento Bar. I hadn't seen the bar before reaching it in the race, and understood that my wife would be there to guide me to my craft as soon as I finished the bike ride. Well, she had been there to meet Keith when he dropped it off, but she wasn't allowed to stay there. Having never so much as touched a surf ski before, I simply could not find it. "It will be in the front row," Keith had assured me. But it wasn't, and for ten to fifteen minutes I went crazy in my search for it. Eventually, almost in tears, I found it among the 700-800 boats, lying fiber to plastic in row after row across the beach. I picked it up and ran with it into the water.

The surf ski was longer, narrower, and lighter than any craft I had ever paddled (19' 6" long, 20" wide, and about 35 lbs). I dropped it on the water and as I got astride it there was a moment of alarming jelly-wobble before I settled into its open well and immediately struck out into the current. I had a lot of catching up to do, but the only craft on the water faster than this Valhalla would be the Necky Phantoms. These were being paddled by elite kayakers like John Weed of Sacramento and Alex Oppedyk from Marin. The only challenge left was taking this knitting needle of a boat through the San Juan Rapid.

What a glorious relief to find the surf ski felt as stable as my own *Arluk II*, and definitely faster; my inner voice reminded me: "Momentum is stability." Away I went to catch and overhaul almost all the 600 cyclists who had ridden past me on the bike section. I had finished the run 90th in a field of 1,500; but I'm not a cyclist at all, and placed in the late 600s when I got off my bike. Then came the down-river race. To get through the San Juan rapid, I lifted my legs out of the well of the surf ski and hung them over the sides. With these stabilizers, the slender surf ski lost some momentum, but we were flushed safely through the rapid. As I went through I saw contestants and kayaks separated from each other all over the place. But in the shallow pool below the rapid there were many volunteers catching and emptying kayaks, and putting their owners back into the race. I got off the surf ski at the end of the down-river dash in the low 100s; and when asked how come I did so poorly in the bike-riding section, I like to joke that I didn't know we were allowed to draft.

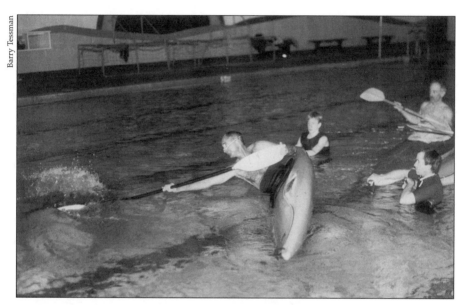

The author teaching the Eskimo roll at the Truckee School pool

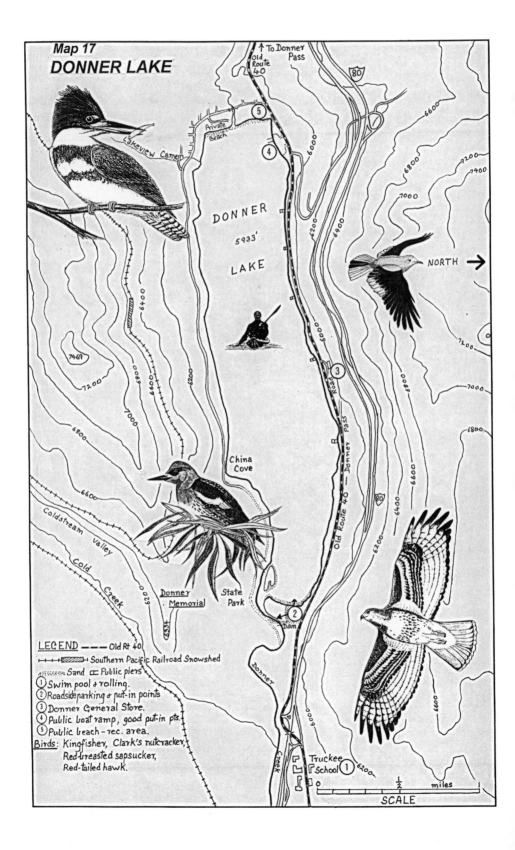

Map 17
DONNER LAKE

To Donner Pass
Old Route 40

80

5

Private Beach

4

D O N N E R

5933'

L A K E

Lakeview Canyon

NORTH →

7469

7200

7000

6800

6600

Coldstream Valley

Cold Creek

6200

6534

China Cove

Donner Memorial

State Park

Old Route 40 — Donner Pass Road

80

Donner

Dam

2

3

6000

6200

6400

6600

6800

7000

7200

7400

7000

7200

6800

6600

6400

6200

6000

Donner Creek

Truckee School

1

6200

LEGEND ——— Old Rt 40

Southern Pacific Railroad Snowshed

Sand ⊏ Public piers

① Swim pool & rolling.
② Roadside parking & put-in points
③ Donner General Store.
④ Public boat ramp, good put-in pts.
⑤ Public beach – rec. area.

Birds: Kingfisher, Clark's nutcracker,
Red-breasted sapsucker,
Red-tailed hawk.

0   ½   miles
SCALE

Chapter 11

Donner Lake, Lake Tahoe, Mono Lake, Pyramid Lake

TRIP 21 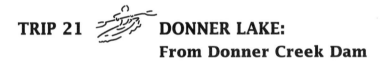 **DONNER LAKE: From Donner Creek Dam**

Type	Length	Map
Easy half-day exploring	6 miles RT to west end	17
Seasonal: best months, May through October		

Summary and Highlights

Donner Lake lies just west of Truckee at 5,933 feet. In summer, as the morning progresses, it becomes a busy recreational lake: at the west end, the public boat ramp is much in demand; the well-maintained, public swimming beach fills up with parents and children; the paddle boats creak and a few jet-skis scream. People fish, sail, and water-ski, but the lake never seems too crowded. It's three miles long and a half-mile wide, and the further east you go, the quieter it becomes. If you drive down to the east end of the lake, the well-shaded woods are cool and pleasant to walk through, and the swimming is unsupervised, yet safe.

An ideal time to use Donner Lake is after driving up from the Bay Area, before you settle down for the evening. If you want real exercise, there's an excellent, 6-mile paddle waiting for you: put in at the east end and go to the west end and back. For local accommodations, there's the Sierra Club's Claire

Tappaan Lodge on Old Route 40 (916) 426-3632, or the Alpine Skills International lodge at the head of Donner Pass (916) 426-9108. And, at the east end of Donner Lake, there is a camping area in Donner Memorial State Park (916) 582-7892.

How to Get There

For the scenic route, take Donner Pass Road off Highway 80 at the SODA SPRINGS NORDEN exit. Drive 3.8 miles to Donner Pass, beyond Sugar Bowl Ski Area on your right, immediately followed by Donner Ski Ranch (the best, little, downhill ski area in California) on your left. As you go over the pass, Alpine Skills International (ASI) is on your right, and you cross the Pacific Crest Trail for hikers—you can clearly see the trail on the left side of the road.

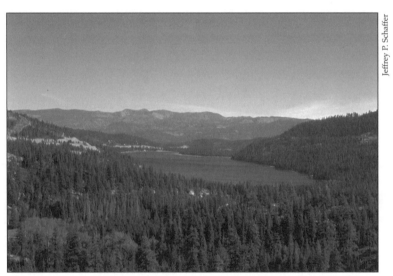

Jeffrey P. Schaffer

An impressive view of Donner Lake looking east from Old Route 40 at Donner Pass

Drive down the pass onto the bridge (over nothing but space) with its scenic overlook of Donner Lake. It is a great view, with Donner Peak, 8,019 feet, to the right. As you go downhill, leaving the overlook, the best-known Donner Pass climbing routes are on a cliff face to your right. After 3.1 miles from the top of the pass, you reach Donner Lake. Stay on Donner Pass Road for another 3 miles beside the lake to a sign, TAHOE DONNER MARINA.

Only a few yards beyond it, a narrow footpath entrance through a low, wooden hurdle fence admits you to the trails of Donner Memorial State Park. There is free, roadside parking by the fence. You may carry your kayak or canoe over the 2-foot fence and follow the path for 100 yards to a small, concrete bridge over a creek. This is Donner Creek, which flows from Donner Lake into the Truckee River. The official entrance to the park, for vehicle parking and the visitor center, is 0.2 mile farther, but you cannot put in from there.

Using Highway 80, instead of the scenic route, going east take the first Truckee exit and turn right to double back along Old Route 40. This will bring you directly to the Donner Memorial State Park entrance; 0.2 mile farther brings you to the free, roadside parking in front of Tahoe Donner Marina. There is no fee for boating from here.

Trip Description

To the right of the bridge, over Donner Creek there is an ideal pool for putting-in to start your trip with a delightful 0.25 mile paddle, upstream, through the woods and into the lake. The dam at the bridge is just below where you put in, and it regulates the top 12 feet of water in Donner Lake released every summer to permit farming between Truckee and Reno. In the recent drought years there had been considerable legal debate about the rights to those 12 critical feet of water. In the summer of 1997, after three successive years of ample snowfall, the argument was quietly shelved.

The creek's banks above the dam are beautifully shaded and clear of undergrowth for a quarter mile before you come to a sandbar, with 2.75 miles of the lake's open water beyond it and with a consistent half-mile width. While in this pleasant, backwater creek you have totally calm, clear water—ideal for canoeing, practicing rolling, or introducing a friend to kayaking. American mergansers breed here, and you are likely to meet up with females, throughout the summer, usually with a flotilla of young. The magnificent, black and white male birds, with their scarlet saw-bills, disappear early in the summer, having no parental duties to detain them.

There is a lot of vocal activity in the woods around you. Steller's jay has a wide vocabulary and an opinion to broadcast on everything. You may hear three species of woodpeckers: hairy, downy, and orange-shafted flicker. All of them fly over the creek from time to time. There will be ground squirrels and chipmunks on the banks; but the most vivid sighting, if you are lucky, will be a western tanager. The male bird is brilliant—about 7 inches long—with a red head, bright yellow body, and black wings and tail. It also has one yellow and one white bar across its black wings. It is often seen in these woods, discreetly followed by the much less vivid, yellow-green female.

When you cross the sandbar into the broadwater of the lake the contrast is considerable. By noon there is always a breeze coming from the west which can build into a wind by mid-afternoon. On the open lake, if you are not a strong paddler, and particularly if you are in a canoe, it is wise to paddle close to shore. You can follow the wooded banks on either the north or south shore of the lake, and on the north shore there are plenty of public places to take

out. The south shore, however, is almost entirely private, and though unpost-
ed it is jealously guarded, so that you take out on that side only in emergency.

If you are a strong paddler, paddling the middle of the lake to the broad,
sandy beach of the west end's public recreation area, 2.75 miles ahead, is fine;
but pay attention because small, fast boats are scudding around the lake,
often towing unpredictable things like inner tubes or water-skis. When starting a water-ski run, a red flag is held aloft in the cockpit of the speed boat—
which then accelerates rapidly. Often, the towed skier fails to get up into a
skiing mode, and the tow boat promptly stops. While all this is going on, an
osprey or occasionally a golden eagle may fly over. What do they make of the
disturbance down below?

As you head west, the Pacific Crest dips to Donner Pass on the right. You
can see the pass, a small saddle, clearly defined along the ridge. If you've read
the book, *The Donner Party*, you can't help recalling that although this pass
was waiting for them, dead ahead, the snow was so deep that the struggling
emigrants turned southwest into a kinder looking canyon. This put them on
the steep, southeast flank of Mt. Judah, in what we now call Lakeview

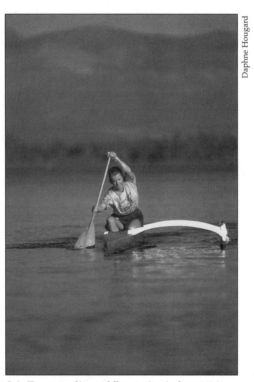

Daphne Hougard

*Jojo Toppner, elite paddler, trains in her outrig-
ger canoe on Donner Lake*

Canyon, where they couldn't recover from their mistake. Then, above you to your left, you become aware, when a train comes through, of the tunnels and the escarpment so harshly built with Chinese labor. After the intrepid early settlers had made it to the West Coast, the railroad through the pass became the critical supporting link.

———— ⚜ ————

I lived at Soda Springs for eight years, and used Donner Lake a lot in the summer. One day, when I was putting in from the open beach, in the northeast corner of the lake, close to the Donner Creek put-in point, there was a strong onshore breeze coming straight down the lake from the west. I saw a man and a small boy in a green canoe, crossing the lake, about 100 yards offshore. Neither one was wearing a life jacket, and the father (I assumed this relationship) was doing the paddling, however ineptly, while his son was right up in the bow.

Canoes carry a lot of wind, and this one was carrying all it could by crossing the wind's path. Small waves were kicking up, and I was anticipating a good, 3-mile workout up into the wind with a great payoff on the return trip. Just as I was launching off the beach, a sudden blast of wind tipped the canoe over. I saw two orange life jackets bouncing around with the whitecaps, and then two, yelling heads apart from the life jackets and making no effort to stay with the canoe.

I shoved myself forward off the sand, and yelled very loudly, "Stay with the boat!" I could see, as I paddled out to them, that they were merely staying afloat and not swimming in any direction. As soon as I was close to the little boy, I told him to hang on to the back of my kayak and stay behind it. Then I turned my attention, and the kayak, toward dad. He was swimming about as well as he'd been paddling, and without giving him a chance to grab at the kayak, I said, "If you stop swimming, you can stand up."

To his great surprise, giving it a try, he found himself standing chest high in the choppy water. "We have to get the boat back," he gasped. But, I told him that it wasn't necessary. I could see the canoe was being blown to the beach, so I yelled, "The boat will put itself on the beach before you."

I towed the little boy, who seemed to be in good shape, and on our way in he spotted the wooden paddle; we changed course a bit so that he could pick it up. When we regrouped on the beach, the little boy thanked me, but his father offered no thanks. All he said was, "How much does a boat like yours cost?"

———— ⚜ ————

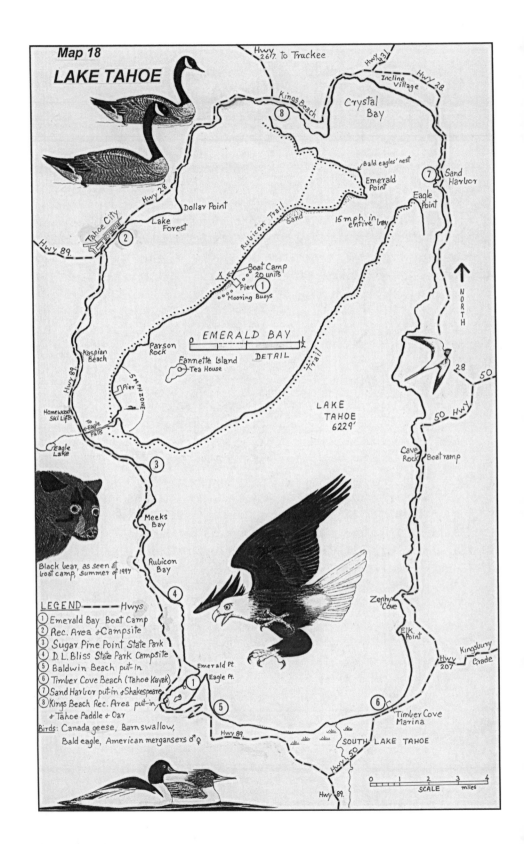

Map 18
LAKE TAHOE

Hwy 267 to Truckee

Hwy 431

Incline Village

Hwy 28

Kings Beach

Crystal Bay

⑧

Bald eagles' nest

Emerald Point

⑦ Sand Harbor

Eagle Point

Hwy 28

Dollar Point

Lake Forest

Tahoe City

Hwy 89

②

Rubicon Trail

Sand

15 m.p.h. in entire bay

Boat Camp 20 units

Pier

Mooring Buoys

①

EMERALD BAY   0 ½

DETAIL

Parson Rock

Kaspian Beach

Fannette Island
Tea House

Rubicon Trail

LAKE TAHOE 6229'

5 M.P.H. ZONE

Pier

Hwy 89

Homewood Ski Lifts

To Eagle Falls

Eagle Lake

③

NORTH

28   50

50 HWY

Cave Rock   Boat ramp

Meeks Bay

Rubicon Bay

Black bear, as seen at boat camp, summer of 1997

④

Zephyr Cove

Elk Point

Kingsbury Grade

Hwy 207

LEGEND ———— Hwys
① Emerald Bay Boat Camp
② Rec. Area & Campsite
③ Sugar Pine Point State Park
④ D. L. Bliss State Park Campsite
⑤ Baldwin Beach put-in
⑥ Timber Cove Beach (Tahoe Kayak)
⑦ Sand Harbor put-in & Shakespeare
⑧ Kings Beach Rec. Area put-in
   & Tahoe Paddle & Oar
Birds: Canada geese, Barn swallow,
   Bald eagle, American mergansers ♂♀

Emerald Pt
Eagle Pt.

①

⑤

Hwy 89

⑥

Timber Cove Marina

SOUTH LAKE TAHOE

Hwy 50

Hwy 89

0 1 2 3 4
SCALE   miles

TRIP 22   LAKE TAHOE:
Sugar Pine Point to Emerald Bay

Type	Length	Map
Moderate full day	14 miles RT	18
Easy overnight	14 miles RT to Boat Camp	18

Seasonal: best months, May through October

Summary and Highlights

Lake Tahoe's perimeter roads add up to 72 miles on my odometer. Since the roads stay close to the water almost all the way, except in the northeast corner of the lake, they outline a large body of water. It is one of the deepest, cleanest, and most easily accessible recreational lakes in North America. In the early mornings it is usually as still as a mill pond, but as the day develops, motorboating alone is enough to generate water disturbance all along the more popular shores. However, there is a lot of space on this lake and there are many quiet areas. Lake Tahoe is magnificently surrounded by mountains from 8 to 10,000 feet high, and it can become a turbulent lake. Many people enjoy second homes here, while others stay in hotels, motels, and lodges, mostly concentrated on the north shore at Incline Village, Kings Beach, and Tahoe City, or concentrated on the gambling shore in South Lake Tahoe.

The lake is 12 miles wide and 22 miles long, with a shoreline of approximately 72 miles. Its average depth is 989 feet, and its deepest point is 1,645 feet. The total surface area is 191 square miles, and the average temperature of the water in August varies between 65 and 70 degrees. Its most famous fish is a trout called the Mackinaw; and you can kayak here year round, if you are hardy.

In terms of the civilized use of the lake, its beaches, and the entertainments available, the Shakespeare "Theater on the Beach," on the north shore at Sand Harbor, tops my list. At the bottom of the list is the stretch of road, "gasping gorge," between the towering walls of Harvey's and Harrah's in South Lake Tahoe. Here you can actually see the pollution haze of this area from far away.

How to Get There

Take the LAKE TAHOE 89 SOUTH exit off Highway 80. Route 89 follows the Truckee River. In 7.5 miles you pass the Squaw Valley turnoff on your right. At

1.5 miles after the Squaw Valley road, the turnoff for Alpine Meadows Road crosses the Truckee River, on your right. The River Ranch Motel, take-out point for all the river rafts coming down from Tahoe City, is on this corner.

There is a bike path between you and the river for the next 3.5 miles to Tahoe City. You see the "Truckee River green" color in some of the deeper pools interspersed along this slow-flowing, Class 1, reach of the river. Throughout the summer, rubber rafts will be floating by; fly-fishers will be casting when they can between the drifting rafters; and bikers and bladers will be cruising by. As you enter Tahoe City, a huge Safeway is on your left and a bronze statue of three Mackinaw trout is on your right. You turn right in front of the statue on West Lake Drive, and follow the sign for EMERALD BAY. This route takes you around the west shore of Lake Tahoe to Highway 50, where it enters South Lake Tahoe.

Circling the Lake

In order to give an overview of the kayaking opportunities around the shores of Lake Tahoe, this section describes the put-in points that are not too complicated to approach, and are in the public domain. There are many of them dispersed around the lake. Some have camping facilities, and one is an environmental campsite in Emerald Bay, which can only be approached for camping from the water. Hikers may walk in to it but may not use it overnight. The mileage for the circling of the lake starts from the Mackinaw statue in Tahoe City and goes counter-clockwise in three sections. This allows drivers coming into the circuit from Route 50 and Route 28 to start their mileage at zero from their point of entry on the counter-clockwise circuit. All the roadside put-in points described are suitable for a day trip of exploration along the well-sheltered shores of the lake. Do not to leave vehicles parked overnight in places that are not designated parking areas.

Going south on Route 89, at 4.4 miles you could put in at Kaspian Beach, by the signed LAKE TAHOE BASIN PICNIC GROUND, with free, roadside parking. At 6.2 miles, Homewood Ski Area is on your right, with their parking lot at roadside. Directly opposite their parking lot, a narrow, unnamed road leads down to the water. You can offload here and then park your car on the Homewood side of the road.

After Tahoma at 9.4 miles, the entrance to SUGAR PINE POINT STATE PARK CAMPGROUND is on your right. For reservations (800) 444-7275. The lakeside entrance to SUGAR PINE POINT STATE PARK (916) 525-7982, is on your left at 10 miles. It is open from 6 A.M. to sunset. I think that it is the outstanding state park on this side of Lake Tahoe; it has a good picnic area, swimming area, and nature center with a book shop. It can be the put-in point for a day trip, or an overnight trip to Emerald Bay. If you need overnight parking, you can offload your kayak or canoe and carry it 85 yards downhill, to the water here. You

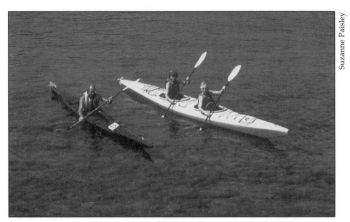

Carol Jeneid and Mary O'Brian with the author after winning their classes in the Lake Tahoe Outrigger Criterion—Canoe and Kayak Classic

will then have to park your car 0.6 mile farther north, at Sugar Pine Point Park Campground. You may leave a car in the extra parking lot at this campground for as long as two weeks. Some people do this, and use Emerald Bay Boat Camp as their base from which to explore the whole lake by kayak.

In 11 miles (1 mile south of Sugar Pine Point State Park), there is a very busy campsite on your left. This is MEEKS BAY NATIONAL FOREST CAMPGROUND BEACH. It costs $14/night and, in summer months mid-week chances of getting a site are quite good. The beach is close, though out of sight from the road. I do not like the overcrowding of the campsite, its closeness to the road, or the lack of security.

The next major park is the D. L. BLISS STATE PARK, 16.6 miles south of Tahoe City (916) 525-7277. This is another well-run park, with swimming, picnicking, and camping. You can use this one as an overnight base from which to kayak, or for a day trip. At 18.6 miles, there is a fine view down into Emerald Bay from the Vikingsholm Parking Lot, and at 21 miles, EMERALD BAY STATE PARK— EAGLE POINT CAMPGROUND is on your left. This is a very good campground for trailers, with a lot of space between sites. But the entire campground is high above Emerald Bay, and it would not be a place from which to kayak.

Just south of Eagle Point Campground, 23.8 miles from Tahoe City, you come to BALDWIN BEACH. It doesn't look promising from the roadside, but it's ideal in terms of parking close to the water and carrying your kayak straight onto the sand beach. It's open 7 A.M. to dusk, from Memorial day through mid-September. For the $3 fee, it is the least complicated put-in point on the west shore. There are two more kayaking beaches, VALHALLA BEACH, at 26 miles, and POPE BEACH, at 27 miles. At 29.5 miles in South Lake Tahoe, Route 89 intersects with Highway 50. Turn left at the light for LAKE TAHOE NEVADA.

Head east from Route 89 onto Highway 50, with your mileage at zero. In 2.5 miles the TAHOE STATE RECREATION AREA and El Dorado Beach will be on your left. Reservations may be made from seven months to one day ahead of use, through Destinet (800) 444-7275. This isn't a quiet campsite; you are barely off Highway 50. Closer to both money and smog, at 3.9 miles TIMBER COVE MARINA is on your left, and behind the lodge there is a very pleasant public beach, the largest on the south shore, from which you can put in. There is also a commercial kayaking operation called Kayak Tahoe (916) 544-2011, from which you can rent or buy kayaks, take lessons, or go on guided tours, including one to Emerald Bay.

Continuing east, a half mile from Timber Cove, the road to Heavenly Valley Ski Area is on your right; and at 4.4 miles, you pass at your peril between the walls of Harvey's and Harrah's. If you make it through that area, at 7.5 miles you can turn left at the traffic lights, off Highway 50, for ELK POINT. A half mile down this road you will come to a campground called NEVADA BEACH CAMP (800) 280-2267. This is a large, full-service campground, with a fine sand beach from which to put in. It's open mid-May through mid-October for camping, $16/site. Day parking is $3.

Leaving Elk Point behind, going north on Highway 50 at 10.7 miles, a ramp leads down to an area called CAVE ROCK, just before the Cave Rock Tunnel. You are in for a nice surprise because what looks at first sight to be a boat ramp for power boats only, with rip-rap rocks all around the shore, is deceptive. At the back of the parking lot, and not visible until you are right on it, is a delightful little sandy beach. It is just perfect for putting in on the east shore. In mid-summer, you'll have to arrive early to use Cave Rock, but it's worth it. You put your $5 fee into the box provided. At 16.2 miles, you reach SPOONER JUNCTION, where Route 28 meets Highway 50.

Start your mileage from Spooner Junction and head east for Incline Village on Route 28. At 3 miles, you come to SECRET HARBOR, which is part of the LAKE TAHOE NEVADA STATE PARK. Here there is good swimming, kayaking, and hiking, with three campsites for walk-in campers only. At 7.4 miles, SAND HARBOR RECREATION AREA is on your left, where there is the Shakespeare Theater and a fine beach for swimming. But to launch any boat, you have to continue 200 yards past the entrance to the park and use the designated boat-launching area.

At State Line you cross into California, and at 17.5 miles, you are in Kings Beach. The KINGS BEACH STATE RECREATIONAL AREA is on your left, with free parking and direct access to a large beach. It is from this beach that the Hawaiian Classic Outrigger Criterion takes place each year on Labor Day. Down the road, 0.1 mile, on your right, is Tahoe Paddle & Oar (916) 581-3029, owned and operated by Phil Segal. It has its rental and on-water facility two blocks down the road, at the North Tahoe Beach Center. They specialize in kayaking the north shore of Lake Tahoe, with guided tours, rentals, and instruction. They offer a special trip to Sand Harbor in Nevada on their pontoon boat, to explore the area by kayak when you get there.

Near Tahoe City, at 25.1 miles, a sign reads, LAKE FOREST—PUBLIC PARK, indicating another recreation area where you can put in. Finally, 1 mile farther, just as you are driving into Tahoe City, at 26.1 miles, a sign on your left says, TAHOE STATE RECREATION AREA AND CAMPSITE.

Of all the places identified as put-in points around Lake Tahoe, I think, for day use, SUGAR PINE POINT STATE PARK, D. L. BLISS STATE PARK, and BALDWIN BEACH on the west shore; TIMBER COVE on the south shore; NEVADA BEACH CAMP and CAVE ROCK on the east shore; and KINGS BEACH on the north shore are the most convenient. All these put-in points are numbered on the map.

Trip Description

An overnight trip at Boat Camp, a site in Emerald Bay specially maintained for boating campers only, is an excellent Tahoe trip. The choice of Sugar Pine Point State Park as a starting point was based on three factors. First, it provides a decent mileage by kayak to Boat Camp—12 miles, measured by road, but less by kayak. Second, it avoids paying for two campsites while sleeping at only one. Third, it starts out from a well laid out and attractive park—an excellent place for bird watching when you're not boating. I have seen three species of flycatcher, and a seldom seen hermit warbler, within fifteen minutes, in the upper canopy of the pine trees.

Having reached the park via the route already described in the previous section, put your $5 in the envelope provided and drive on 100 yards to a NO ENTRY sign in front of you. Turn right at this sign and follow the dirt road south for 0.1 mile. The lake is below you on your left, and there are numerous, small pull outs for parking. Choose one directly above the lakeside boathouse. Carry all your gear down to the beach; and, for a day trip to Boat Camp or any other place you may leave your car where it is. But, if you are going to stay out overnight, drive your car out of this park, 0.6 mile north, and leave it in the overflow parking section of Sugar Pine Point State Park Campground.

If you are starting in the early morning, the water is likely to be calm; and there is a little sand-grit beach on either side of the boathouse, for putting in. As you leave the shore you will be impressed with the size of the lake and how far away everything, except the tall pine trees on your right, seems to be. Since you are heading south, the sun will be on your left, or just over your left shoulder. The extraordinary clarity of the water, as you move around a few subsurface boulders, will immediately surprise you. Aim for a red buoy ahead of you; and keep in mind that when you move any distance away from Lake Tahoe's shores you are in deep water—very deep water.

Emerald Bay is 12 miles from Sugar Pine Point by road. Yet, within minutes of setting out, you'll round a corner and see Meeks Bay, a deep indentation in the shoreline, with a nice looking sand beach. Now you'll realize you can cut straight across the bay to the next point. If you keep doing this from headland to headland, you can probably halve the distance from Sugar Pine Point to Emerald Bay. Once you leave the red buoy behind, the sense of distance is similar to being out at sea on a calm day. Everything on shore is a continuum of vague images that are hard to recognize, except for the sand beaches and headlands. This trip is a fine opportunity to experience a combination of solitude and safety—hard to come by so close to civilization.

Unless the wind is up and the water rough, going from headland to headland, along this reach of the lake to Emerald Bay, is the way to go. In this way, 12 miles will become 7. The south point of Meeks Bay, which you are now aiming for, is the north point of Rubicon Bay. That bay looks like one, long, open, 2-mile curve, seen from a half-mile out on the water, with Rubicon Peak towering 9,183 feet behind it. In fact, it's two bays of almost equal size, separated by a prominent beach. You'll see some cliffs at the start of the second part of the bay, and, if you are interested in rock climbing, you may want to check them out. They are an interesting 80 to 90 feet of Class 5 climbing on a series of good slabs. They'd be hard to climb from the water because there's isn't any beach, so you'd probably rappel down to start a route. If you go in close, you may see a few people walking a trail high above you, and you will see a steel cable handrail above the cliffs. There must be a designated trail up there.

As the sun moves ahead of your left shoulder, you'll start to see mirages of distant pine trees that come right out into the lake—many miles it seems—from the heavily forested shore. It becomes impossible, looking ahead, to assess the distance to anything. Only the shoreline to your right makes any recognizable sense. No matter how hard you try, you won't be able to tell where the real trees end and the mirage trees begin.

One distant landmark stands out: Heavenly Valley's ski runs are very obvious, and you know they converge above South Lake Tahoe. If you make a 360 degree turn, you can take in a panoptical view of what is really so special about Lake Tahoe, the unbroken ring of high mountains entirely surrounding it. South, behind Heavenly, there is a superb saddle between two peaks well over 10,000 feet; and, if you follow the mountains east, your eyes will bring you northeast to the 10,778-foot summit of Mt. Rose. Now you need to keep track of where you are by looking ahead to your right; there, you can see Rubicon Point coming up, and the sand beach and campground of the D. L. Bliss State Park, tucked into the south corner of Rubicon Bay.

After Rubicon Point, the headland that comes sharply into focus is Eagle Point, the southern headland of Emerald Bay. Even 1 mile away you can't visually distinguish the mouth of this narrow bay; only one thing gives it away. For some time now a large number of big, powerful boats have been roaring past Eagle Point and disappearing without a trace. These boats are passing between Eagle and Emerald points, and disappearing into the narrow sleeve of Emerald Bay.

As you get closer to Eagle Point, you can see the "eagles' nest" that a pair of bald eagles built here. It is at the top of a tall pine tree with a magnificent view of the lake and Emerald Bay. As you approach the nest for a better view, your kayak will be tossed around by the turbulence created by the boats charging in and out of the bay. Apparently, this precious bay, and a quick trip around Fannette Island, is the thing to do if you have a big boat. A kayaker can get out of the way by hugging the north shore, where there are shallows, with rocks and deciduous trees forming their own islands and creating calm water. You can follow these shallows right into the bay, where you will find a boat dock and a little bit of sand, just enough to beach, at Boat Camp.

Boat Camp has well-sheltered campsites, and in the woods to your right as you approach it, you will hear and may see bright-yellow, evening grosbeaks and western wood pewee flycatchers. On the water there will almost certainly be Lake Tahoe's diving duck, the American merganser; and throughout

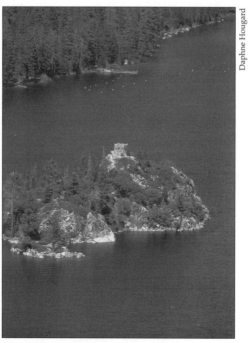

Daphne Hougard

Emerald Bay's Fannette Island with Boat Camp's jetty in the background

June, July, and August, whole families of these birds will be cruising around and sunning themselves on the rocks. You'll also hear Clark's nutcrackers and, with any luck, see them. They move around a lot.

There are toilets and firewood provided at Boat Camp, but drinking water is your own responsibility: passing the lake-water through a purifier is good enough for me. Campsites are available on a first-come, first-served basis; even in midsummer, you will get a site if you arrive late in the afternoon Sunday through Thursday (that's my opinion, not a fact). On Fridays and Saturdays, campsites fill up quickly. You are allowed to stay two weeks for a fee of $10 for each day's occupancy of one campsite. You can definitely fish for your supper from here, with a chance of catching kokanee, one of the Alaskan salmon stocked in the lake. The secret is a live minnow, with your bait swimming so that it has about 3 feet of line from it to your lead, which is on the bottom. Richard Scholk, the camp host when I came through, does very well with this technique, fishing from his canoe in depths ranging from 30 to 100 feet.

I made this trip in mid-August, arriving at Boat Camp at noon on a Sunday, to find a choice of sites available and a riddle to solve. Long before I got under the "eagles' nest" at Eagle Point, I could see the "eagles" all right, but only by half their scientific name. It is a fine nest, and its occupant when I arrived was not an eagle but my old friend Pandion haliaeetus, *the osprey. It turned out that the real eagles' nest (that of the bald eagle,* Haliaeetus leucocephalus: *meaning "the white-headed sea eagle) is on the north side of Emerald Point, and though I paddled around to see these huge birds, I found the nest, but no eagles were present. What the osprey and the bald eagle (both are fish-eating birds) share in their scientific name is recognition that both were considered "sea eagles" by the early taxonomists who named them. But* Pandion *(King of Athens), in the osprey's name, was a "flight of mythological exuberance" on the part of the taxonomist, Savigny.*

There was only one problem with this beautiful campsite; it was the non-stop shuttle of big boats being driven through Emerald Bay at exactly 15 mph, to the letter of the law. The worst speed you can drive these boats, because it sets up maximum wake, is 10 to 15 mph. If ever a public boating locale called for 5 mph limit, Emerald Bay is it. On weekends, there are scores of large powerboats running around — wrecking a wonderful haven by turning it into a boating bedlam. "Paddles, oars, or sails," should be the order for this lovely bay. Fannette of the Island, whoever she was, must be seasick in her grave every time one of these marauding stinkpots comes cruising by.

A question, someone who doesn't know Lake Tahoe, or the Emerald Bay boating situation, has asked me, is this, "Is it worth being out there with all those boats charging around?" I answered that question 27 years ago in a classroom at Boston University, when I was teaching there. A professor in the psychology department had invited me to meet his students, and suggested that I let them choose a topic for discussion. "Would you talk about existential ontology?" one student asked. And, in a flash, I said, "Yes, I'd like to do that." So I spoke about kayaking, solo, on open water that is also being used by powerboats. This was something I'd done many times off Lordship, in the broad and boat-busy mouth of the Housatonic River.

My theme was simple: the ontological concept of being a kayaker, self-propelled in a boat hand-built by oneself (I built my first kayak—with adult help—when I was twelve years old), rather than having a power boat and operating it at great expense. That, plus the existential reward of being totally self-sufficient, rather than dependent on a huge motor that demands a consistent, expensive fuel supply. When the fuel line gets clogged, or the fuel runs out, or your motor breaks down, you can't drive your prized possession. I told the class, "The ability to pace yourself, and especially the ability to save yourself, when in danger, instead of calling out for help, is what really counts. This is the kayakers gestalt." And I went on to explain that doing an Eskimo roll with your kayak, having been knocked upside down by a wave, is obviously a utilitarian move. It is also an existential move, if only because it prompts you to take pleasure in your existence; it gives a boost to your morale as well as bringing you back to the surface. "That's a mystical moment: when movement and mind are perfectly matched, and you solve the problem of being underwater, upside down, locked in your kayak."

This was my theme, and all I can say of this class is that the same professor asked me back to repeat it, and some of his class came kayaking with me. We kayaked the entire Hudson River, from its first navigable source in the Adirondacks all the way to the Battery in Manhattan. It took 26 days to cover 318 miles, and among the things we studied were forestry, geology, and the Hudson River School of Painting. The students kept journals and earned six credits toward graduation, while their adventure was featured in The New York Times. *So that's what I'm doing out there—wherever I am—exploring the existential opportunities of life—in my kayak—with or without the powerboats. As for the waves these big boat-toys make in the water, they are something to play with. The waves they make become surf—existential fuel for an ontologist.*

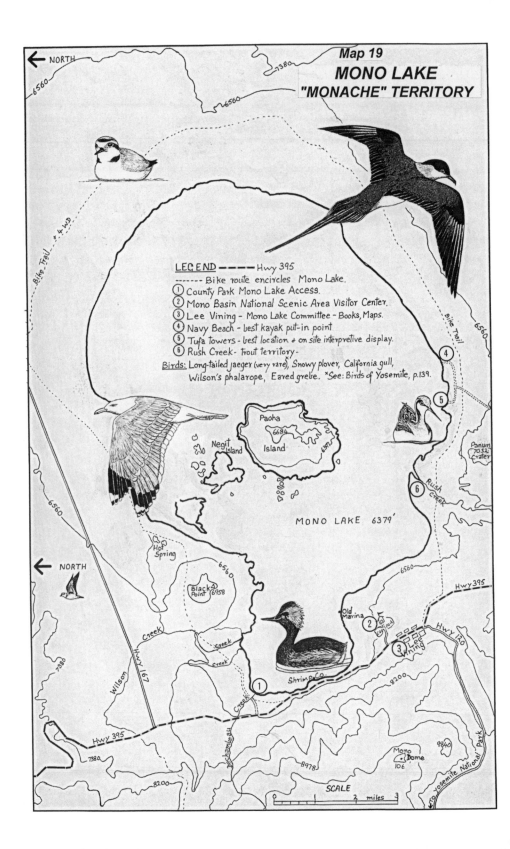

Map 19

MONO LAKE
"MONACHE" TERRITORY

NORTH

6560

7380

6560

6560

Bike Trail - 4-w.D

Bike Trail

6560

LEGEND ————— Hwy 395

------- Bike route encircles Mono Lake.
① County Park Mono Lake Access.
② Mono Basin National Scenic Area Visitor Center.
③ Lee Vining - Mono Lake Committee - Books, Maps.
④ Navy Beach - best kayak put-in point
⑤ Tufa towers - best location & on site interpretive display.
⑥ Rush Creek- Trout territory-
<u>Birds:</u> Long-tailed jaeger (very rare), Snowy plover, California gull,
Wilson's phalarope, Eared grebe. *See: Birds of Yosemite, p.139.

④

⑤

Panum
7034
Crater

Paoha
6684
Island

Negit
Island

6391

Rush
Creek

⑥

MONO LAKE 6379'

6560

NORTH

Hot
Spring

6560

Black
Point 6958

Hwy 395

Hwy 167

Creek

Creek

Creek

Creek

Wilson

Old
Marina

②

③ Lee
Vining

Hwy 395

Hwy 120

8200

① Shrimp Co.

Mechanic St.

7380

8978

8200

Mono
Dome
106

9840

to Yosemite National Park

SCALE
0   1   2   miles   3

TRIP 23   MONO LAKE:
Navy Beach to Country Park

Type	Length	Map
Strenuous full day	20 miles RT	19
Moderate full day	14 miles RT to Old Marina	19
Easy day shuttle	10 miles one way to County Park	19

Seasonal: harsh winter environment; best months, May through October.

Summary and Highlights

Mono Lake is one of the oldest lakes—over 700,000 years old—in North America. It is 8 miles long, north to south, and 13 miles wide. It covers 60 square miles and has two large islands, Negit and Paoha, that are the special breeding territory of the California gull. It is famous for its salinity (2.5 times more salty than the sea) and its tufa towers. These mysterious-looking towers have risen above the water level only because of the loss in the lake's depth over the past 50 years; they are nature's response to the salty water in the lake being tickled by naturally carbonated water from under the lake. The mingling of carbonates in the lake water with calcium in the spring water results in a deposit of calcium carbonate, which builds up into a tufa tower.

It is a desert lake, at an elevation approaching 6,379 feet, set off by a border of magnificent mountain peaks, rising to 13,000 feet. Just south of the lake, is the youngest volcanic mountain range in North America, the Mono Craters. The youngest of these popped up only 600 years ago. Both islands on the lake are volcanic, and Paoha is only 300 years old. From the scenic overlook at 8,000 feet as you approach from the north on Route 395, Mono Lake is a breathtaking sight.

Special Advice

The highlights of Mono Lake will be best enjoyed if, as you approach Lee Vining, you orient yourself to the area at the Scenic Area Visitor Center & Reserve Office (760) 647-3044. There are no developed campsites around Mono Lake. Free, environmental camping is allowed around the lake, above its 1941 high water level, but only after reading and signing the Letter of Authorization for Camping. *You must comply with this authorization at the Visitor Center before setting out to camp.* Also check out the Mono Lake Committee store in Lee Vining (760) 647-6595 for advice, maps, and guidebooks, before you set out. The Mono Lake Committee, founded by the late

David Gaines, who has done the most to save the lake from being consumed by ever-thirsty L.A.

If you are going to spend much time kayaking on this saline, desert lake, you must carry a good supply of drinking water; and extra water for washing yourself salt-free after kayaking or swimming. Because of the severity of the lake's conditions—heat and capsizing winds are two threats—if you are going far, particularly if you are alone, someone should know how long you intend to be out there. And you should check in with that person when you come out.

How to Get There

From Sparks or Reno, Nevada, head south on Route 395, off Interstate 80. From Highway 50, at South Lake Tahoe, take Route 207 east for Minden and Gardnerville, over the Kingsbury Grade. This is a steep, winding, mountain climb with a long descent to a pastoral plain, where cows graze and white-faced ibis breed. In 10.7 miles, having reached the bottom of the grade, turn left for Route 395, and at 13.7 miles turn right. In another 3.1 miles, your road will join Route 395, going south, and take you all the way to Lee Vining, near Mono Lake.

Along the way you'll probably see magpies, eating road kills or balancing on roadside fences; and at 40 miles from South Lake Tahoe you'll come to Topaz Lake, where Canada geese live in large numbers. White pelicans stop off here, in the spring and fall, on their way to and from their breeding grounds. Highway 108 to Sonora Pass will be on your right at 67 miles, and you'll reach Bridgeport at 84 miles. Here, you can get 24-hour, emergency medical care, should you need it.

As you make the long climb to an elevation of 8,138 feet, approaching the overlook to Mono Lake, you will have several miles in which to enjoy some high, saw-toothed peaks. Then, between you and these mountain ridges, there are generous folds in the open hills, with long groves of aspen trees. They offer immense relief to the severity of the land surrounding them; and in the fall, their beauty is unrivaled.

At 98 miles, you drop over the crest of the pass and have to pull off the road to catch your breath. Here, you will see all of what John Muir saw when he first looked down into the Mono Basin: "hot deserts bordered by snow-laden mountains, cinders and ashes . . . frost and fire working together in the making of beauty." How sad to think that the fire in the opal of this particular lake was nearly extinguished by human greed; it was nearly extinguished by people who never saw the lake, but took the water from creeks and streams that flow into it, without which the lake could not survive.

At 104 miles, in the Mono Lake Basin, you'll see a sign for COUNTY PARK MONO LAKE ACCESS. If you turn left on this road, in a half mile, you'll come to a small park with toilet facilities. You may not want to detour now, but don't leave Mono Lake without visiting this park. This is where you'll leave your shuttle vehicle if you do the 10-mile trip from Navy Beach. It is the oasis on the shoreline of the lake; a lush, wild garden, to be visited preferably at dawn, or soon after, so that you may enjoy the incredible variety of birds singing. Their music ranges from the nuptial drumming of "pond-snipe," diving from the sky to issue their reverberating vows, to the "careless happiness" of the meadowlark, as it, "keeps on giving its song a try." (That's Walt Whitman, again.)

At 108 miles, just short of Lee Vining, on your left you will see the Scenic Area Visitor Center & Reservation Office from which the use and protection of Mono Lake is supervised. Here you can get authorization for camping from your kayak or from your vehicle. There is a 4WD road around the east half of the lake, and you are permitted to camp from your vehicle along this route. You may also camp on the islands after the gull breeding season is over—August 1 is the official date.

After the visitor center, Lee Vining and the Mono Lake Committee store are just ahead. It's a small town with several motels, one good American-style diner, coffee shops, a large grocery store, and a gas station. Tioga Lodge on Mono Lake (888) 647-6423 where Ansel Adams used to stay, has several cozy cabins, and a restaurant, 2.5 miles north of Lee Vining, on Route 395. Walter

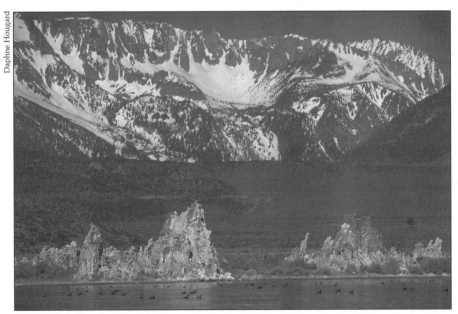

10,000-foot mountains are an impressive background for Mono Lake's eared grebes and their tufa towers

and LaJuana Vint have rescued and rebuilt this lodge, which had been closed for many years. It is much quieter here than in the town, and close to County Park for a dawn chorus visit.

To reach the put-in point at Navy Beach, starting from the Mono Lake Committee store front in Lee Vining, go south on Route 395 for 5.3 miles, and turn east on Route 120. Follow this road and, at 10 miles, turn left onto an unpaved road for South Tufa Area & Navy Beach. At 10.8 miles, the road splits; turn left for South Tufa Area (with interpretive displays of area animals, plants and minerals). For Navy Beach, continue ahead for another 0.5 mile. At 11.3 miles you arrive at a small parking lot, 40 yards from the water. Note one important sign: when ospreys are nesting on the tufa column directly ahead, as you look at the lake, do not approach their nesting site in your kayak. Too many disturbances may result in the nests being abandoned.

Trip Description

On a desert lake like Mono, it matters that you start early and paddle with the sun at your back because the light is so intense. So, start out early from Navy Beach, with the sun behind you, to explore the shoreline as far as County Park, on the northwest corner of the lake, 10 miles away. A slow paddle there with a good lunch break will put the sun in the right place for the return trip. For the best bird watching by kayak, August and September are the months of choice; that's when the phalaropes arrive, followed by huge numbers of eared grebes that come here at this time of year. You can check ahead with the Mono Lake Committee to find out when the birds are coming in (619) 647-6595. The phalaropes, which are shorebirds, fly in and stay long enough to engorge on brine flies, gaining twice their body weight on arrival, to sustain them on their 3,000-mile flight to wintering quarters in Argentina. The grebes are a diving bird, more interested in the brine shrimp.

Millions of little black brine flies may be forming a collar around the very edge of the littoral wherever you put in. They are absolutely harmless and will stay down by your ankles. There is no need to swat at them or kick them. They, and the brine shrimp, are the most valuable creatures in the food chain of the lake. They are the fuel for the migrating birds who migrate here.

On your left as you leave Navy Beach, you can see "Tufa City," officially designated the South Tufa Area. It is one of the favorite areas of the lake for phalaropes, and it has the most concentrated area of tufa towers. These towers are very fragile and soft, though they look like concrete from a distance. Don't allow your kayak to hit them or scrape against them; those that are subsurface but close enough to scrape, are clearly visible in the water. As you navigate between the towers you will see the most beautiful of swallows, the violet-green swallow, flying around the tufas and perching on them. The phalaropes, feeding, and spinning around like wind-up toys while at it, will

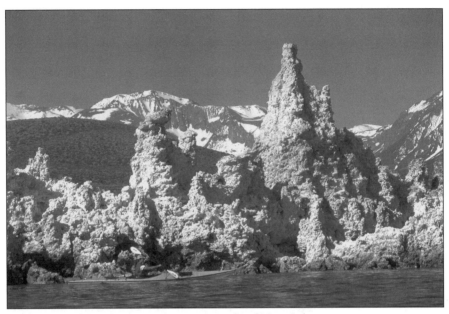

Daphne Hougard glides among the towering tufas of Mono Lake

barely move aside as you glide along. Killdeer plovers will run along the littoral and make a fuss as you come by; avocets, with their rust-colored necks and faces, may appear; and you will always be aware of the California gulls in the air.

After 2.5 miles, there is a point in the shoreline, and around it you can see and hear a great deal of gull activity. As you come up to the point you can tuck yourself right into the shore and peek around it. When you do you will get quite a surprise. There will be hundreds of gulls, that you hadn't been able to see, sitting on the water and, splashing about as if they were in the public baths, getting rid of the salt in their system. This is where historic Rush Creek, the creek that was really put on trial in court, fans out into a broad delta and ends its journey in Mono Lake. It is pouring fresh, effervescent water into the briny lake, and the gulls love it. They aren't alone. Caspian terns and ospreys fish here, too. Remember, there are no fish of any kind in Mono Lake because it's too salty, but here there are trout. Also, county regulations require you to stay out of the Rush Creek Delta.

This delta is the destination of fresh water from Grant Lake, combined with water from Parker Lake and Walker Lake, tumbling down their respective creeks into Rush Creek. It was here, in 1984, that a fly-fishing realtor, Dick Dahlgren, found a few brown trout barely surviving; he took their plight to a Los Angeles attorney, Barret McInerney, and an Inyo County judge issued a temporary restraining order. Judge Donald Chapman then ordered Los

Angeles water-hogging administrators to release more water into Rush Creek. The incident marked the turning of the tide in Mono Lake's favor; and in 1994 the case to save Mono Lake was resolved. Enjoy this place.

After Rush Creek there's a bay you can cut across in 2 miles, or follow the shoreline for 3, to reach the next tufa town. A mile farther on you come to another fresh water inlet to the lake, Lee Vining Creek. Now you have to pass around a curving headland, which brings you, in 1 mile, to the Old Marina Site and another tufa town. You have paddled at least 7 miles, and this may be as far as you want to go in a day—if you have been paddling slowly and absorbing all there is to see. It's worth remembering that very strong winds rise up, without warning on this lake, particularly in the afternoon. Stay close to shore, and don't commit yourself to traveling over open water unless conditions are stable.

If you feel like going beyond the Old Marina, there's a nice little bay behind the tufas, and it's one of the favorite areas for Wilson's phalaropes. In another 2 miles you'll be seeing green marshland and rushes, instead of barren soil, along the shore, and you'll come to the only sign of any industry, apart from tourism, to be found on Mono Lake. There is a small shrimping industry, a company called High Sierra Brine Shrimp owned by Tim Hansen, that hauls out about 100 tons of brine shrimp per year. His are the only motorized boats you are likely to see on Mono Lake, and occasionally they put out to rescue kayakers who have run into trouble. The brine shrimp end up in pet shops, after being processed to become tropical fish food.

From late April through October, the brine shrimp are clearly visible in the water; in fact, you can catch them in your hands. They are somewhat translucent, about a half-inch long, and they are edible. But it is the brine flies that have the more fascinating life cycle. The adult flies crawl down the exposed tufas to sub-merge themselves under water and lay eggs. But they need air; and so, as they go below, their hairy bodies and waxy coating allows them to create a bubble of air in which they are encased. They can stay under for 15 minutes in this condition to lay eggs. Tiny larvae emerge from the eggs, 1-2 millimeters long, and feed on algae growing on mud and rocks. As they grow they have legs, the last two of which have claws with which to clamp themselves onto the underside of a tufa. This prevents the wave action in the water from washing them ashore. Finally, the larval skin hardens to form a pupa case, and inside each case the larva becomes a brine fly. In about two weeks, the adult fly pops the front of its pupa case and floats up to the surface. As soon as its wings are dry, it joins the hordes of flies that make a black collar around the rim of the lake.

If you paddle as far as the County Park, at the end of this route, you'll be rewarded by the lush vegetation and see many birds that you won't see along the predominantly arid shoreline. You will also find shade. There will be warblers, hummingbirds, and that beauty, the yellow-headed blackbird. Restrooms are available at the top of the boardwalk, which comes right down to the water's edge. You have covered 10 miles by now and, unless you have placed a second vehicle in the parking lot here, you have a long haul back to Navy Beach.

Mono Lake takes its name from the Yokuts word for the "brine fly." The lake's early inhabitants, the Kuzedika Paiutes, were called Monache *("people of the lake of the fly") by the neighboring Yokuts, because they harvested the pupae of the alkali flies that abound in the lake. Brine flies and their pupae are the primary food source for five species of birds that come here specifically to live off them: the California gull and the snowy plover, both of which breed here; Wilson's and red-necked phalaropes; and eared grebes. There are another 80 migratory species that include brine flies in their diet. So, Mono Lake has a very special role in the life cycle of a large number of birds. Visually, of course, it is one of the rarest sights in North America, and would not be so if it were allowed to become a salt pan.*

No wonder that it took an ornithologist, the late David Gaines of Lee Vining, to lead the fight that saved the lake. For 50 years, the Los Angeles Department of Water and Power abducted Mono Lake's vital fresh water resource from the five precious streams that provide it. Only in 1994, after 16 years of bitter court action, did sanity prevail. It was prompted by a fisherman and a judge, both of whom revered rainbow trout, though by that time, the lake had lost 55 feet of its depth and had doubled its salinity.

I see that David Gaines, with whom I shared my rare sightings at the lake, included my adult long-tailed jaeger in his book on the Birds of Yosemite and the East Slope. *In August of 1983, my wife, Carol, and I had a fabulous view of this oceanic gull marauder that may have followed a flock of California gulls inland from the coast. It flew about 25 feet above our heads as we ate our lunch, and it looked down at us as if curious. Minutes later, we saw it again, this time tearing around the onshore tufas, chasing a little kestrel falcon that had caught something.*

In May, 1997, Carol and I were kayaking past the South Tufa Area, watching the Brewer's blackbirds that were everywhere on the towers. They were making quite a racket, and one male bird was perched atop the tallest tufa of them all. In a breathtaking second, a male prairie falcon swept in, low over the lake, and threw itself up at the tufa on which the blackbird was holding forth so cheerfully. The poor blackbird never knew what hit it. It was quite simply snatched from the high perch of its happiness to be the falcon's next meal.

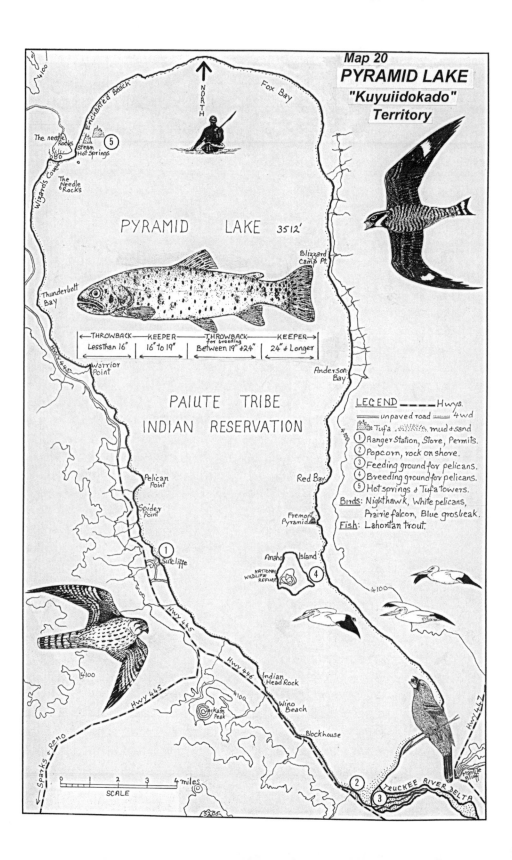

Map 20
PYRAMID LAKE
"Kuyuiidokado"
Territory

NORTH

Fox Bay

Enchanted Beach

The needle Rocks

⑤ Steam Hot Springs

Wizards Cove

The Needle Rocks

PYRAMID LAKE 3512'

Blizzard Camp Pt.

Thunderbolt Bay

THROWBACK	KEEPER	THROWBACK for breeding	KEEPER
Less than 16"	16" to 19"	Between 19" & 24"	24" & Longer

Warrior Point

Anderson Bay

PAIUTE TRIBE
INDIAN RESERVATION

Pelican Point

Red Bay

Spidey Point

Fremont Pyramid

Sutcliffe ①

Anaho Island

NATIONAL WILDLIFE REFUGE

④

Hwy 445

Hwy 446

Indian Head Rock

Jackass Peak

Wino Beach

Blockhouse

TRUCKEE RIVER DELTA

Hwy 447

Middle Bluff

Sparks & Reno

0   1   2   3   4 miles
SCALE

LEGEND ——— Hwys.
═══ unpaved road ┈┈┈ 4wd
🏛 Tufa ⋯⋯ mud & sand
① Ranger Station, Store, Permits.
② Popcorn, rock on shore.
③ Feeding ground for pelicans.
④ Breeding ground for pelicans.
⑤ Hot springs & Tufa towers.
Birds: Nighthawk, White pelicans, Prairie falcon, Blue grosbeak.
Fish: Lahontan trout.

4100

5285

TRIP 24   PYRAMID LAKE:
Sutcliffe to the Truckee River Delta

Type	Length	Map
Moderate overnight	20 miles RT to Popcorn, plus 2–4 miles of delta exploration	20

Seasonal: harsh winter environment; best months, May through October.

Summary and Highlights

Pyramid Lake lies, north to south, in a semi-desert region of Nevada, 32 miles northeast of Reno. It is 30 miles long, 12 miles wide at its broadest, and 5 miles wide at its narrower, southerly end. It survives in the Great Lahontan Basin, at 3,512 feet, surrounded by mountains rising to 8,000 feet. (20,000 years ago it was just one of the deep pockets in a huge basin of water, called Lake Lahontan.) Most of the lake is about 300 feet deep, and it has a shallow shoreline with beaches of fine gravel that makes it easy to put in and haul out a kayak. Like Mono Lake, this lake is saline (but much less so than Mono) because it has no outlet; and it is the destination of the Truckee River, which flows out of Lake Tahoe, traveling 72 miles, via Reno, to get here.

The people of Pyramid Lake, the Northern Paiute, settled here about 500 years ago, and called themselves *Kuyuiidokado*, "the eaters of the *Cui ui*" (pronounced cooey-ooey). They spent a lot of time in and on the water, fishing for this large, endangered species of carp-like fish, which lives only in this lake. Like the Miwok of Tomales Bay they didn't make kayaks, but they made rafts of dry, pithy tules, tied in bundles, which they maneuvered in and out of the reed-beds. Apart from fishing for the magnificent Lahontan trout and *Cui ui*, rabbit skins and white pelican skins were among the other resources to be taken from around the lake. From these, clothes and blankets were made; and today both jack rabbits and white pelicans are still abundant. The surrounding desert is filled with wildlife: flowers, horned and collared lizards, weasels, coyotes, cottontails and jack rabbits. Silver fox, antelope and mule deer live here, and birds are everywhere. All you have to do is get to the Truckee delta by kayak, tuck yourself into the surrounding scrub, be patient, and watch. Everything will come to you.

Special Advice

Pyramid Lake is a Paiute Tribal Territory; you must check in at the Sutcliffe Ranger Station, or at the Pyramid Lake Visitor Center and Store on Highway

445, for $5 camping permits and fishing permits. Camping is allowed all around the lake, except for the northern end, where the tufas and hot springs are. We have vandalism to thank for this recent restriction. In spite of that, the lake is one of the most magnificent inland waters to explore; but, before you do so, time spent in the excellent museum, at the visitor center, will be time well spent. Cars can be left at the marina parking area at Sutcliffe, or parked anywhere along the shoreline where you are camping. While it is usually very calm in the mornings, violent winds can spring up without notice later in the day. The west shore is typically the lee shore, and you should not be far from it if weather conditions deteriorate.

How to Get There

Follow Interstate 80 to Sparks, Nevada. Take the PYRAMID WAY EXIT 18, in the shadow of The Nugget gambling casino, onto Pyramid Way (Highway 445). This route will take you all the way to Pyramid Lake. Resetting your odometer at Exit 18, the National Wild Horse and Burro Center will be on your right at 18.5 miles. You may see several hundred wild horses, if there has recently been a wild-horse round up or sale. Every effort is made to find ranch homes for the wild horses when they are auctioned.

At 29 miles, you come to a scenic overlook on your right, with a great view of Pyramid Lake. Across the water, 5 miles away, you can see Anaho Island, where the white pelicans breed, and the much smaller Pyramid Island from which the lake takes its name. At 29.7 miles, your road swings north and starts to run parallel to the lake, toward Sutcliffe. At 32.5 miles, you turn right on Sutcliffe Drive, and follow it to the left as it curves along the shoreline. When you come to the bar and casino at 33.2 miles, turn right toward the waterfront. Turn left at the STORE—GAS sign to reach all facilities; at 33.5 miles: RANGER STATION—PYRAMID LAKE VISITOR CENTER & PYRAMID LAKE MARINA. Permits are sold from the store in the visitor center, year round, well into the evening, or in the ranger station from 9 a.m to 5 p.m. Food, bottled water, and maps are available in the store, and there are bathrooms in the museum section of the building. When you have obtained your camping-boating permit ($5/day), you can head around the lake in either direction to camp from your car on the beaches. There is a small marina and harbor in front of the main facilities in Sutcliffe; you may safely leave your vehicle there while you take off for your trip.

Trip Description

On the trip I describe you start out at the marina and head 10 miles south, down to a beach known as Popcorn. There is a large rock at the roadside, above this beach, which looks like a gigantic piece of popcorn. There is also a single toilet, close to the beach in the parking area below Popcorn. You may camp and rest up in Popcorn in preparation for your Truckee River Delta

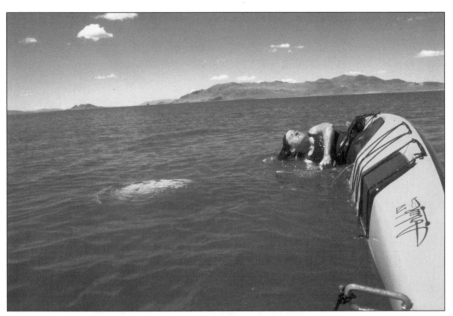

Daphne Hougard practices a version of the Eskimo roll in Pyramid Lake—with Anaho Island and the Fremont Pyramid in the distance

exploration, or you may start hiking toward the delta and follow its southerly bank. The delta is shallow with swiftly flowing water, so that a reconnaissance on foot is a good idea. On the 10-mile paddle down to Popcorn, you can haul out almost anywhere; there are many small coves with easy, sloping beaches along the way. You'll meet a few cormorants, western grebes and white pelicans (there are only white pelicans on this lake), and you'll see few motorized boats heading this far down the lake. Surrounded by a ring of mountains set well back from the lake—the view from the water is so impressive—you feel exhilarated to be here.

Pyramid Lake has been evaporating at the rate of one foot per year, for many years. This is due to its vast surface exposure to the sun, and the abducted inflow of fresh water from the Truckee River since the construction of the Marble Bluff Dam. The effect is visible as you watch the shoreline; you can see stages of the lake's depletion by both the sculpted design of the beaches, and the wide margin between water and scrub vegetation. You may smell something not unlike sewage as you get close to Popcorn, but it is only sulfur coming from warm springs along the shore. It is perfectly safe to swim in the lake, even though you may find floating algae makes it less appealing. (In 1995, I requested a scientific check of the water in the area of Popcorn. The authorities checked it and gave me a clean report.) You can taste enough salt in the water to know that you wouldn't want to drink it.

There's a nice little beach, facing southeast, just before Popcorn, and it's a good spot for the night. You will be facing the delta that is the reason for your coming this way. From April through August, you will see as many as 2,000 white pelicans, in the air and etched in long lines in the shallows, only a half mile in front of you. They are feeding here, where all the nutrients brought into the lake from the Truckee River have created the area in which fish thrive. The pelicans and the double-crested cormorants fish side by side; both of them are at the top of their food chains.

An initial investigation of the delta on foot has the advantage in that instead of battling the swift-flowing water for control of your kayak, both hands are free for using your binoculars. If you want to see everything that's in the scrub, and behind the wonderful, 10-foot tamarisks, as well as what's on the water, go on foot and spend a whole day immersed in the world of the horned lark, the lazuli bunting, and the yellow-headed blackbird. It's very hot in there, so take something with you that you can set up for shade. (I always take an umbrella.)

If you'd rather spend your time hanging out with the pelicans, then the kayak is the answer. Take your time approaching them; don't go too close because there's no need to. They will come drifting toward you. Some of them will be traveling backwards because there is no need not to; they have no enemies to escape. In fact, they have so much discretionary time that they can play. Your rule of approach should be clear: the moment you see signs of unrest among them, stop.

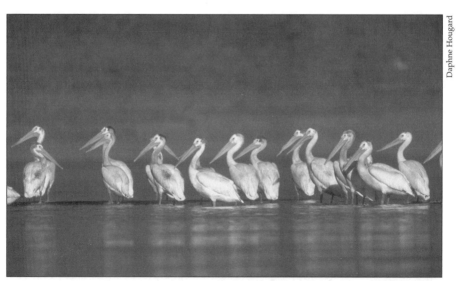

A colony of white pelicans breeds at Pyramid Lake while others stopover from Salt Lake City

This route and the project of exploring the delta is ideal for a group of students. In 1996, I published an article about kayaking and bird watching at Pyramid Lake in Sea Kayaker Magazine *called, "A Few Days in Paradise." As soon as it came out, I got a phone call from a teacher, Buck Wales, at the Thacher School, in Ojai, Southern California, suggesting that I join his group of kayakers. He was about to lead ten students on a five-day kayaking trip to Arizona; but, having read my piece, he wanted to try Pyramid Lake instead. So I drove up there and met his gang at Sutcliffe, intending simply to help get them started.*

It was already October and the pelicans were long gone, except for the odd straggler. Buck's gang had slept out on the beach the night before we were due to meet, and I was looking everywhere for them, an hour after dawn. As I was approaching the water, I walked into one of those occurrences that are part of my life, but always seem unique. I found myself in a clearing, and standing there in front of me on the ground—perhaps 30 yards away—facing each other in some sort of petulant stand-off were three birds of prey.

A very big hawk—a whole two feet of him—with bright chestnut-feathered shoulders, black wings and a big, pallid tail, dominated the scene. It had chestnut trousers, too, with lots of black barring. It just stood there, round shouldered, with its tail well clear of the ground, glowering at something between it and the other two birds. These two were much smaller than the hawk, and one was bigger than the other, though neither one could be called small. They were both khaki brown, with dark mottling on their backs and folded wings, and their fronts were dusty white with heavy spotting. What really excited me were the dark mustachal markings behind and under their heavy eyes. I was able to observe them because they all seemed immobilized by my sudden appearance; besides, there was this thing on the ground between them, which all were loath to leave.

The big ferugious hawk broke the spell: lumbering off, beating with disdain its powerful wings that spanned five feet. And it showed me the whiteness of its broad tail. This was too much for the pair of prairie falcons. As the bigger, female bird led their rapid withdrawal, I was able to walk up to the freshly killed jack rabbit that one of these three had killed. Which one? I still wonder.

That took place an hour after dawn. So, welcome to Pyramid Lake in the off-season. In the spring, which is when I most like to be there, the pelicans are arriving in large numbers, every day. Gliding in groups of 30, 50, sometimes more than 100, they construct elegant formations, winding like white ribbons around the mountains as they slowly decide where to land. And they actually do "the wave," just as you see spectators in a stadium who coordinate rising and sitting in order to create a wave effect. It occurs to me that these pelicans invented the wave. By late May there will be 2,000 of them here; such magnificent birds, whose wingspans exceed all others, matching the California condors' 109-inch spans. Their massive bills look like huge, pale carrots.

But there are flowers, too, and in the spring their dominant color is yellow. All over the west shore are large monkey flowers that look like long-stemmed pansies; balsam roots, like large, floppy dandelions; cinquefoils, like buttercups; blazing stars that look exactly like that; and stickleaves that look like oaktree leaves. There are yellow pimpernels, instead of scarlet, and wild violets that look just like violets but are yellow. Then there are mauve and purple flowers, too: dramatic sego lilies, wild peonies, and showy milkweed; and one flower that can't be left unnamed, the dramatic, purple-blue wild iris.

In 1995, I found a bird breeding at Pyramid Lake that no one, on record, had seen there before. I checked this carefully with an ornithologist from the University of Nevada at Reno, someone who monitors the area. I had hidden my kayak in the tamarisks and purple grass alongside the main channel of the delta, and set myself up comfortably to see what might come by. A pretty song, that I half-recognized but couldn't quite identify, filtered its way into my mind. I heard the song again and began to search for its owner. Two blackbirds were waving around in the wind, clinging to the top of their tamarisk, and facing them from another tall stem of the same kind, was the singer. I knew at once I was seeing something rare, if only because I'd been coming here for so many years and never seen this bird.

I was now standing clear of all cover, and the heat was like a furnace under the blazing Nevada sun. Even the bird was panting, its powerful beak agape. It had to be open because it had something black and round in its oversized beak, possibly a beetle. Using my powerful binoculars, I could see every detail of its brilliant plumage. It was the size of a street sparrow, but so richly indigo, cobalt, and chalk blue, with all these blues fluctuating as it swayed in the sunlight at the top of its tamarisk that I could hardly believe what I was seeing. Its folded wings were black, with two outrageously orange-rust wing bars, like half-chevrons proclaiming its rank.

My very first thought was that it was a lazuli bunting, but it was the variance from this bird's song—a song I knew—that had tipped me off. I had never seen it anywhere before, because I'd never been near its territory in the southern states. And now I knew that I had found a blue grosbeak. A few moments later, lower down on the same tamarisk, I found his partner. She was delightfully discreet compared with her brilliant mate. She had a lovely, buff-olive bloom all over, with soft nuances of her partner's blue and orange-rust; and she had the same black eyes, black legs, and over-sized beak.

The "cerulean-blue bird" is the meaning of this bunting's scientific name, Guiraca caerulea, *and it could not be more appropriate. As I had it framed in the magnified circle of my binoculars, there were black-tipped white wings gliding— in slow motion—it seemed, through the background of the image. I wondered where in the world one can possibly see white angels and brilliant blue grosbeaks simultaneously through one lens? Only in Paradise, or at Pyramid Lake.*

Appendix 1—Kayaking Outfitters & Trip Leaders

TOMALES BAY:

Blue Waters, P.O. Box 983, 12938 Sir Francis Drake Blvd., Inverness 94937, (415) 669-2600. Rentals, tours, instruction.

Tamal Saka, P.O. Box 833, Marshall 94937, (415) 663-1743. Rentals, tours , instruction.

BOLINAS LAGOON:

Off The Beach—Ocean Kayaks Ltd., P.O. Box 885, Stinson Beach 94970, (415) 868-9445. Kayak sales, rentals, instruction, tours.

Stinson Beach Health Club and Kayaks, P.O. Box 635, Stinson Beach 94970, (415) 868-2739. Kayak sales, rentals, instruction, tours.

Paddlebirding, P.O. Box 1060, Stinson Beach 94970, (415) 868-2302. Birdwatching and kayaking instruction.

SAN FRANCISCO BAY:

Sea Trek, Sausalito, Schoonmaker Harbor, kayaking site (415) 332-4465. Sea Trek reservations, P.O. Box 561, Woodacre 94973, (415) 488-1000. Rentals, tours, instruction, expeditions.

California Canoe and Kayak, Jack London Square, 409 Water Street, Oakland 94607, (510) 893-7833. Sales of all classes of kayaks and canoes, equipment, clothing, books, videos; rentals, instruction, tours, expeditions.

R.E.I., 1338 San Pablo Avenue, Berkeley 94702, (510) 527-4140. Sales of kayaks and canoes, books, videos and all outdoor clothing and camping gear.

HALF MOON BAY:

Tsunami Rangers, P.O. Box 339, Moss Beach 94038, (650) 728-5118. Sales of custom made Tsunami kayaks, advanced sea kayaking instruction, and instruction videos.

California Canoe and Kayak, Pillar Point Harbor, P.O. Box 394, El Granada 94018, (650) 728-1803. Primarily rentals and instruction—particularly surfing skills; some equipment sales.

SANTA CRUZ:

The Kayak Connection, above small yacht harbor, 413 Lake Avenue, Santa Cruz 95062, (408) 479-1121. Kayak sales, clothing and accessories, books, videos. Rentals, tours, instruction, expeditions.

Adventure Sports, 303 Potrero Street, Santa Cruz 95060, (408) 458-3648. Kayak sales of all varieties, rentals, instruction, tours, expeditions; clothing, accessories, books, videos.

Venture Quest, 125 Beach Street, Santa Cruz 95060, (408) 427-2267. Kayak sales, accessories, rentals, instruction, tours, expeditions.

MOSS LANDING:

The Kayak Connection, Elkhorn Yacht Club, Highway 1, Moss Landing 95039, (408) 724-5692. Kayak sales, clothing and accessories, books, videos. Rentals for tours and instruction on Elkhorn Slough.

MONTEREY BAY:

Monterey Bay Kayaks, Monterey State Beach, 693 Del Monte Avenue, Monterey 93940, (408) 373-5357. Kayak sales (Necky and Current Designs specialists), clothing, accessories, books, videos. Rentals, instruction, tours.

SACRAMENTO:

California Canoe and Kayak, American River Parkway, Lower Sunrise River Access, 11257 Bridge Street, Rancho Cordova 95670, (916) 631-1400. Sales of all classes of kayaks and canoes, equipment,clothing, books, videos; rentals, instruction, tours, expeditions.

LAKE TAHOE, SOUTH SHORE:

Kayak Tahoe, Timber Cove Marina, P.O. Box 11129, South Lake Tahoe 96155, (916) 544-2011. Rentals, instruction, tours off Timber Cove beach.

NORTH SHORE:

Tahoe Paddle and Oar, P.O. Box 7212, Tahoe City 96145, (916) 581-3029. Kayak and canoe sales, accessories, books and videos. Rentals, instruction, tours.

MONO LAKE:

Mono Lake Committee, P.O. Box 29, Highway 395 at Third Street, Lee Vining 93541, (760) 647-6595. Good book shop. Expert, interpretive tours by canoe to the South Tufa Area, summer and early fall, weekends only.

Appendix 2—Suggested Books, Videos, and Supplies

KAYAKING:

TIDELOG: Graphic Almanac for Northern California—*including San Francisco Bay and Delta, south to Monterey, and north to the Nehalem River, Oregon.* Pacific Publishers, Box 408, Bolinas CA 94924, $10.

California Coastal Access Guide, University of California Press. Price varies: $17.95 at CCK, up to $25 in some stores.

California Boating and Water Sports, Tom Stienstra. Foghorn Press, $19.95.

The Essential Sea Kayaker, David Seidman. McGraw Hill, $19.95

The Basic Essentials of Sea Kayaking, Mike Wyatt. ICS Books, $5.95

Kayaking Made Easy—*A manual for beginners,* Dennis Stuhaug. Globe Pequot Press, $17.95.

The Complete Book Of Sea Kayaking, Derek C. Hutchinson. Globe Pequot Press, $19.95

The Bombproof Roll and Beyond, Paul Dutky. Menasha Ridge Press, $19.95

Learning The (Pawlata) Eskimo Roll With Carol, Michael Jeneid. Personal Performance Programs, $5.

BIRD FIELD IDENTIFICATION GUIDES:

Field Guide to the Birds of North America, National Geographic Society. This one is bigger than a pocket book, but excellent. $21.

A Guide to Field Identification—Birds of North America, artist Arthur Singer. Golden Press,$14. (This is my preferred pocket book.)

Peterson's Field Guide to Birds of North America, Roger Tory Peterson. Houghton Mifflin, $17.95

SEA KAYAKING VIDEOS:

Sea Kayaking—getting started—produced by Larry Holman. $29.95.

Adventures of the Tsunami Rangers and Tsunami instruction videos—Contact Eric Soares at (650) 727-5118, $25.00

Surf Zone Kayaking: Contact John Lull, P.O. Box 564, El Granada, CA 94018, $25.00

INEXPENSIVE BINOCULARS FOR BIRD WATCHING:

Under $200: 8X40 (8X is magnification, 40mm is the diameter of the object lens) is my suggestion. The more powerful your glasses, the more wobble in the image—especially in a kayak. In the $150-200 price range, **Bushnell** binoculars are recommended by the Audubon Society. I do not recommend binoculars below this price range.

Appendix 3—Beaufort Wind Scale

Beaufort Number	Seaman's description of wind	Velocity m.p.h.	Estimating velocities on land	Estimating velocities on sea	Probable mean height of waves	Description of sea
0	Calm	Less than 1	Smoke rises vertically	Sea like a mirror		Calm (glassy)
1	Light Air	1–3	Smoke drifts; wind vanes unmoved	Ripples with the appearance of scales are formed but without foam crests	1/2	Rippled
2	Light breeze	4–7	Wind felt on face; leaves rustle; ordinary vane moved by wind	Small wavelets, still short but more pronounced; crests have a glassy appearance. Perhaps scattered white caps.	1	Smooth
3	Gentle breeze	8–12	Leaves and twigs in constant motion; wind extends light flag.	Large wavelets. Crests begin to break. Foam of glassy appearance. Perhaps scattered white caps.	2-1/2	
4	Moderate breeze	13–18	Raises dust and loose paper; small branches are moved.	Small waves, becoming longer, fairly frequent white caps.	5	Slight
5	Fresh breeze	19–24	Small trees in leaf begin to sway; crested wavelets form on inland water.	Moderate waves, taking a more pronounced long form; many white caps are formed. (Chance of some spray.)	10	Moderate
6	Strong breeze	25–31	Large branches in motion; whistling heard in telegraph wires; umbrellas used with difficulty.	Large waves begin to form; the white foam crests are more extensive everywhere. (Probably some spray.)	15	Rough
7	Moderate gale	32–38	Whole trees in motion; inconvenience felt in walking against wind.	Sea heaps up and white foam from breaking waves begins to be blown in streaks.	20	Very rough
8	Fresh gale	39–46	Breaks twigs off trees; generally impedes progress.	Moderately high waves of greater length; edges of crests break into spindrift. The foam is blown in well-marked streaks along the direction of the wind.	25	High
9	Strong gale	47–54	Slight structural damage occurs.	High waves. Dense streaks of foam along the direction of the wind. Sea begins to roll. Spray may affect visibility.	30	
10	Whole gale	55–63	Trees uprooted; considerable structural damage occurs.	Very high waves with long, overhanging crests. The surface of the sea takes a white appearance.	35	Very high
11	Storm	64–73		The sea is completely covered with long white patches of foam lying along the direction of the wind. Everywhere edges of the wave crests are blown into froth. Visibility affected.	40	
12	Hurricane	74–82		The air is filled with foam and spray. Sea completely white with driving spray; visibility very seriously affected.	45 or more	Phenomenal

Index

About the Author

When I was young, sheer athletic fitness allowed me to participate in events in which I hadn't much skill. Fitness and a burning desire for independence allowed me to make some interesting journeys by kayak, like my solo trip from London to Paris in 1957, to see a friend. The year after this trip, while still in the Royal Marines and with many more ocean miles under my stern, I went back to France in the same kayak. Only this time I had a companion, a little golden hamster. We traveled together, she in her biscuit tin while at sea, from the Royal Navy Gunnery School on Wale Island, in Hampshire, to the white cliffs of Dover, in Kent. Just as he had in '57, Captain Hayes, the Royal Cinque Ports Yacht Club secretary, saw me off from the Dover Harbor beach. He was much less worried about me than he had been the previous year; mainly, I think, because the weather was stable. He didn't know I had a stowaway hamster with me. Six hours and thirty minutes after our departure from Dover Harbor, Hamster and I landed on the sands of Wissant, France, famous as the starting-finishing point for cross-Channel swimmers. It was a slow run compared with the previous year's effort, when

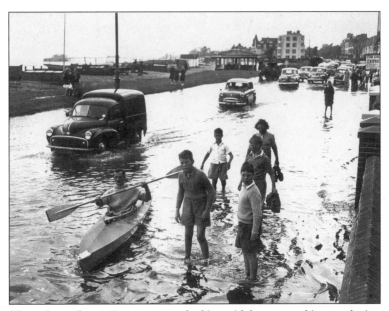

The author—almost 40 years ago, embarking with hamster on his second trip to France—kayaks a flooded street in Worthing, England

there was a Force 4–5 wind on the Beaufort Scale that threw me across the Channel. Hamster made her Channel crossing without being seasick, and from Wissant I walked into Calais for food, leaving her in charge of the kayak. That night we slept on the beach inside my canvas craft. The next morning we took off again, and we were back in Dover Harbor in just over eight hours.

The sea was tediously calm both ways, but entering Dover Harbor was as hard as anything I had done. Hamster and I had drifted way too far east, toward the Goodwin Sands, and I was very tired by the time we reached the English coastline. There were miles of extra slogging to do, into a current that was almost too much for me, and the mole around the harbor was like a chastity belt with the key thrown away. Throughout those extra hours, whenever I thought we couldn't make it, I visualized the statue in Dover, commemorating the Free French Commandos from World War II. It has a memorable inscription, which reads: *"L'audace, encore de l'audace, toujours de l'audace."* ("Courage, more courage, always courage.")

As for Hamster, she was, I think, the first of her kind to have crossed the English Channel by kayak, traveling both ways in two days, back to back. So she was renamed, and became Admiral Hamster because golden hamsters come from Syria, where they speak hamster Arabic. The word "admiral" is a purely Arabic word that does not necessarily denote naval rank; it means "one who commands the sea."

Kayaking entails unavoidable risk that every kayaker assumes and must be aware of and respect. The fact that a trip is described in this book is not a representation that it will be safe for you. Kayaking trips vary greatly in difficulty and in the degree of conditioning and skill one needs to enjoy them safely. On some trips the area may have changed or conditions may have deteriorated since the descriptions were written. Trip conditions change even from day to day, owing to weather and other factors. A trip that is safe on a calm day or for a highly conditioned, experienced, properly equipped kayaker may be completely unsafe for someone else or unsafe under adverse weather conditions.

You can minimize your risks on the water by being knowledgeable, prepared and alert. There is not space in this book for a general treatise on safety on the water, but there are a number of good books and instruction courses on the subject and you should take advantage of them to increase your knowledge. Just as important, you should always be aware of your own limitations and of conditions existing when and where you are kayaking. If conditions are dangerous, or if you're not prepared to deal with them safely, choose a different trip, or don't go at all. It's better to have wasted a drive than to be the subject of a rescue. These warnings are not intended to scare you off the water. However, one element of the beauty, freedom and excitement of kayaking is the presence of risks that do not confront us at home. When you kayak you assume those risks. They can be met safely, but only if you exercise your own independent judgement and common sense. The author and the publisher of this book disclaim any liability or loss resulting from the use of this book.